Medical Information on the Internet

Dedication

To T.H.K.

For Churchill Livingstone

Commissioning Editor: Peter Richardson
Project Controller: Anita Sekhri
Design Direction: Sarah Cape
Marketing Executive: Louise Ashworth

Medical Information on the Internet

A Guide for Health Professionals

Robert Kiley BA (Hons) MSc ALA

Health Sciences Librarian, Frimley Park Hospital NHS Trust, Surrey

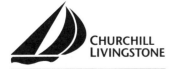

EDINBURGH LONDON NEW YORK PHILADELPHIA SAN FRANCISCO SYDNEY AND TORONTO 1998

CHURCHILL LIVINGSTONE
A Medical Division of Harcourt Brace & Company Limited

First published 1996
Reprinted 1997
Reprinted 1998

ISBN 0443 056994

British Library Cataloguing in Publication Data
A catalogue record for this book is available from
the British Library.

Library of Congress Cataloging in Publication Data
A catalog record for this book is available from
the Library of Congress.

Medical Knowledge is constantly changing. As new
information becomes available, changes in treatment,
procedures, equipment and the use of drugs become
necessary. The editors/authors/contributors and the
publishers have, as far as it is possible, taken care to
ensure that the information given in this text is accurate
and up to date. However, readers are strongly advised to
confirm that the information, especially with regard to
drug usage, complies with the latest legislation and
standards of practice.

The
publisher's
policy is to use
paper manufactured
from sustainable forests

Printed in the USA

Contents

4. The top ten medical resources   43

5. Interactive learning   63

6. E-mail, discussion lists and newsgroups   79

Preface

The Internet is everywhere. If you pick up a newspaper, you will find stories about it. On the radio and television, you are as likely to hear e-mail addresses being cited as contact points, as telephone or fax numbers. Even advertisements, for items as diverse as beer and building societies, now include a reference to the product's presence on the World Wide Web.[1,2]

This interest in the Internet is not restricted to the popular media. Editors of medical journals accept articles about the Internet and welcome correspondence by e-mail; some actually publish via this medium. For example, the *BMJ Classified Section*, probably the most popular medical title in the UK, can now be accessed on the Internet.[3]

Being aware of the Internet, and being able to use it effectively are, however, two very different things. Indeed, in my role as a health sciences librarian I find that though the majority of health professionals have read about the Internet and are enthusiastic about its potential, few have any clear idea of how they can tap into this mass of information to find data relevant to their needs. Addressing this problem is one of the primary themes of this book.

In realising this objective, I have concentrated on providing practical illustrations of how the Internet can be of use to health professionals on a day-to-day basis. For example, though the section on Usenet newsgroups explains what these are, the *focus* of the discussion is, first, about how health professionals can identify newsgroups appropriate to their specific interests; and second, about issues such as how the 'news' can be filtered so that time is not wasted reading irrelevant mailings.

By concentrating on the practical aspects of how health professionals can make best use of the Internet, it is hoped that this book will be of use to both Internet novices and veterans.

One of the problems of writing about the Internet is the danger that it will be out-of-date before it is published. To minimise this risk, this book is complemented by a series of World Wide Web pages through which you can link to the key medical resources. You can also use these pages to e-mail me with comments and suggestions.[4]

The medical and health-related resources available on the Internet are vast. This book will introduce you to some of the key sites, but more importantly it will equip you with the necessary tools for you to undertake your own exploration.

Guildford, Surrey **Robert Kiley**
March 1996

REFERENCES

1 Guinness Home Page:
   http://www.guinness.ie/
2 Nationwide Building Society:
   http://www.nationwide.co.uk/homepage/homepage.htm
3 BMJ Classified:
   http://www.tecc.co.uk/bmj/
4 Churchill Livingstone Medical Information on the Internet
   http://www.churchillmed.com/BOOKS/medinter.html

Acknowledgements

My thanks to:

Caroline Sawers, Assistant Regional Librarian (South Thames West);
Peter Richardson, Director, Health Care Information & Management, Churchill Livingstone;
Dr Soicher, Ophthalmologist, Frimley Park Hospital NHS Trust;
James Gardiner, Demon Internet;
Staff and colleagues at Frimley Park Hospital NHS Trust;
Genevieve Kiley.

I would also like to thank the many people (most of whom I have never met) who took the time and trouble to respond to my requests for information.

March 1996   **Robert Kiley**

About the CD-ROM

Enclosed with this book you will find a free CD-ROM, containing the entire searchable text of the book, together with all the Internet screenshots in colour.

To install the CD, follow the instructions on the disk itself. The CD will work with both PC (Windows) and Macintosh systems.

If you are new to the Internet, you may prefer to read the book first, and then explore the CD. If you are already using the Internet, and are comfortable with CD-ROMs, you may wish to use the book and the CD together from the beginning.

If you do not already have a connection to the Internet through an Internet service provider (see ch. 2), the CD contains the necessary software to connect you via a service provider called Earthlink. However, the CD-ROM will work with any Internet provider, and with a wide range of Web browsers.

In addition, you can use the CD-ROM to connect *directly* to any of the Internet sites mentioned in the book, by double-clicking on the relevant URL (or Internet address) while viewing the text on the CD. To do this, you will need to be connected to the Internet, and to have a World Wide Web browser installed (see ch. 2 for details).

Finally, you can access a home page for the book on Churchill Livingstone's World Wide Web site. The address for the book's home page is:

**http://www.churchillmed.com/BOOKS/
medinter.html**

We hope you enjoy both the book and the accompanying CD-ROM!

1

Why use the Internet?

Box 1.1   Objectives of this book

- Explain in a non-technical fashion how you set about getting your computer connected to the Internet (Ch. 2).

- Demonstrate how you can find information on the Internet *specific* to your needs (Ch. 3).

- Alert you to some of the premier health and medical sites now available on the Internet, and demonstrate how access to these can help you perform your day-to-day clinical work more effectively (Chs. 4, 5).

- Introduce you to some of the key communication services on the Internet and show how these can be used in a practical way (Ch. 6).

- Examine how the Internet is evolving and what impact this will have on the future delivery of health care (Ch. 7).

INTRODUCTION

With many health professionals already experiencing information overload – 'infoglut' – the prospect of accessing the Internet where *more* health resources can be found, may appear somewhat daunting.[1,2,3] This feeling may be further exacerbated by thoughts that getting connected to the Internet and subsequently finding relevant information, are both difficult, time-consuming tasks best left to computer whiz-kids. Indeed, a recent letter to the *BMJ* concluded that:

I have not counted the many hours spent in this exercise but I would advise only serious computer enthusiasts with plenty of spare time to access the Internet from home.[4]

The purpose of this book is to allay these fears, and demonstrate how the Internet is becoming an indispensable tool for today's health professional.

1

To put the book in context though, it is necessary to briefly examine the sources of medical information that can be accessed without connecting to the Internet.

MEDICAL INFORMATION BEFORE THE INTERNET

Historically, medical information has always been well organised. Since 1879, with the launch of *Index Medicus*, health professionals have had access to bibliographic tools that can be used to identify published research. Over the years *Index Medicus* has been joined by other databases such as *Excerpta Medica* and *Psychological Abstracts*. The subsequent publication of these and other databases in an electronic form has made the task of retrieving medical information a quick and relatively painless experience.

Finding research that has proved to be effective has also become easier in recent months with the development of databases of systematic reviews such as the Cochrane Collaboration Database and the NHS Centre for Reviews and Dissemination (NHSCRD).

Consequently, a physician looking for some recent reviews and evidence of effective therapies to manage *Helicobacter pylori* for example, can, with a few keystrokes, find highly relevant publications. Moreover, as the resources cited thus far are available *without* an Internet connection, is there a need for health professionals to get connected? Why this question can be answered with a resounding yes, is discussed below.

THE INTERNET FOR HEALTH PROFESSIONALS

Throughout this book you will find numerous examples that demonstrate why the Internet is so important. Box 1.2 summarises what the Internet provides for health professionals.

Perhaps the best way to demonstrate the potential of the Internet is through an example. Continuing with the *H. pylori* subject search mentioned above, Box 1.3 shows *some* of the sources that can currently be found on the Internet.

This single example demonstrates the range of material that is published on the Internet. In

---

Box 1.2 Reasons for connecting to the Internet

- Current and up-to-date information. Even with today's modern publishing methods it can still take many weeks before research findings submitted for publication find their way into print. It takes even longer for the traditional bibliographic databases to index these items. The Internet, however, enables instant publishing, and instant retrieval.

- Access to **both** traditional and new sources of information. If, for example, you were undertaking research into the aetiology of epiglottitis, you could undertake a search of the MEDLINE database, view a video on how you assess a child with this complaint, and participate in an interactive self-assessment test on this subject (Ch. 5). It should also be noted that the majority of new resources published on the Internet are not available through any other format.

- The functionality to access all resources through one local phone call to your Internet provider (Ch. 2). Before the widespread development of the Internet, if you personally wanted to access a range of resources via your computer and modem, you would need to be prepared to dial a number of information providers, many of whom would not be accessible via a low-cost local telephone number.

- Access to all resources through one piece of software – the World Wide Web browser – thus minimising the time it takes to become 'Internet-literate'.

- The opportunity to discuss medical issues with colleagues and experts from around the world though e-mail, discussion lists and newsgroups.

- The opportunity to pursue your research interests and continuing medical education studies from your own home at a time that is convenient to you.

---

this case at least, not one of these sources would have been found by a traditional trawl through the bibliographic databases.

USING THIS BOOK

A great deal of jargon is associated with the Internet. Whenever possible this will be kept

---

Box 1.3 *Helicobacter pylori* subject search

- A full-text consensus statement from the National Institutes of Health on *H. pylori* in peptic ulcer disease.[5]

- The *Helicobacter pylori* Foundation <u>Home Page</u> where you read about the diagnosis and treatment of the disease, look at a list of the most frequently asked questions and their answers, and participate in a discussion forum (Fig. 1.1).[6]

- A list of all the clinical trials that are currently taking place on *H. pylori*. Each trial cited details its nature and objective, and provides contact names and <u>e-mail addresses</u> where further information can be found.[7]

- A treatment table detailing drug combination and dosage for managing *H. pylori* infections. (Data validated by the American Gastrointestinal Association.[8])

- A true/false self-assessment test on diagnosing *H. pylori* infections.[9]

- A full-text article from the evidence-based medicine journal *Bandolier* on the effectiveness of antibiotic regimens in eradicating *H. pylori* infections (Fig. 1.2).[10]

- Endoscopic views of a man's stomach showing a bleeding duodenal ulcer. From this image you are asked to diagnose the condition, *Helicobacter pylori* gastritis (Fig. 1.3).[11]

---

to an absolute minimum, but when there is no alternative, such terms will be underlined. On the Internet underlining indicates a <u>hypertext</u> link to a related document. In this book the link is to the glossary, which can be found in Appendix E. To ensure that this convention does not cause unnecessary distraction only the *first* occurrence of a glossary term in any chapter is underlined.

Throughout the course of this book you will be introduced to a wide range of health resources available on the Internet. Some will be interactive, such as the *Interactive Patient* where you 'interview' the client in an attempt to diagnose the illness. Some will use multimedia features such as audio and video. Others will simply be text. Whatever the medium, emphasis will be placed on how you can find appropriate information quickly and efficiently.

It should also be noted that the overwhelming majority of Internet resources are available free of charge. Some sites, such as the American Medical Association for example, insist that you complete an on-line registration form before an 'access ID' is granted. However, even in cases such as this, the registration details are only collected to enable the publishers to analyse who is accessing their resource.

Consequently, unless explicitly stated otherwise, all the Internet sites listed in this book are available to any Internet user, free of charge. The only costs you will incur are those levied by your telecommunications and Internet providers.

To help you get a feel of what the Internet looks like, many of the examples cited here will be supported with screen shots. When no screen shot is provided, the full Internet address, known as the <u>uniform resource locator</u> (URL), will be cited. For example, the <u>URL</u> of the American Medical Association is:

http://www.ama-assn.org/

Once your Internet connection is in place (Ch. 2), you can jump directly to any cited resource through your World Wide Web browser. If you use <u>Netscape,</u> the most popular Web browser (Appendix B), this is achieved by mouse-clicking on the File | Open Location option and entering the URL *exactly* as it is shown. As many of the computers that make up the Internet are <u>UNIX</u>-based, the case in which you type the address is significant. In the example given below merely entering BANDOLIER in capital letters will cause your Web browser to report that the file 'cannot be found':

http://www.jr2.ox.ac.uk:80/Bandolier/band12/ b12–2.html ✓

http://www.jr2.ox.ac.uk:80/BANDOLIER/ band12/b12–2.html ✗

However, before you can begin to search for information on the Internet, you need to get your computer hooked up. Chapter 2 looks at how this can be achieved and at what cost.

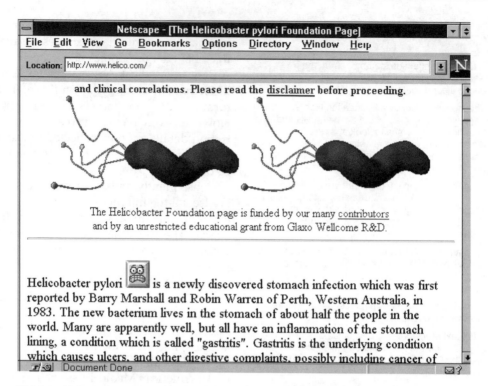

Fig. 1.1 *Helicobacter pylori* Foundation Page

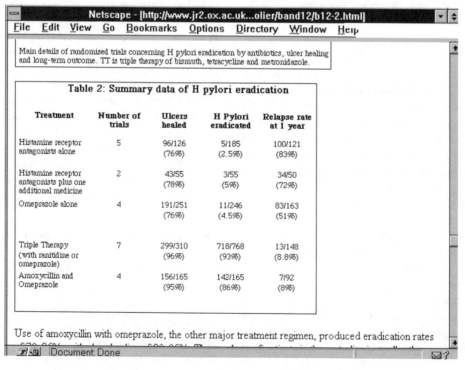

Fig. 1.2 Article from the evidence-based medicine journal, *Bandolier*, on the effectiveness of antibiotic regimens in treating *H. pylori* infections

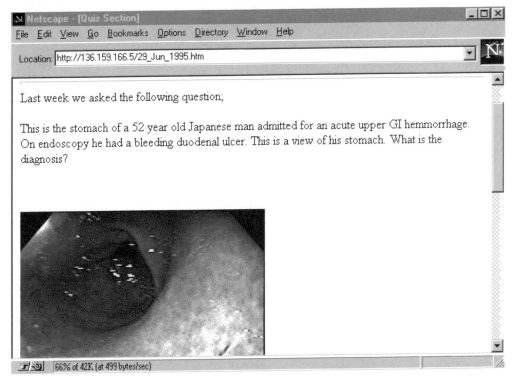

Fig. 1.3 Endoscopic view of a stomach. What is the diagnosis?

REFERENCES AND NOTES

1 Laskin D M Dealing with information overload (editorial). Journal of Oral and Maxillofacial Surgery 1994 52 (7):661
2 Hendee W R Information overload and management in radiology. American Journal of Roentgenology 1991 156 (6):1283–1285
3 Faber R G Information overload (letter). British Medical Journal 1993 307 (6900):383
4 David T J Accessing the Internet is far from easy (letter). British Medical Journal 1996 312:55

5 http://text.nlm.nih.gov/nih/cdc/www/94.html
6 http://www.helico.com/
7 http://www.centerwatch.com/CAT76.HTM
8 http://www.vianet.net.au/~bjmrshll/table1.htm
9 http://uhs.bsd.uchicago.edu/uhs/topics/helico.tf.html
10 http://www.jr2.ox.ac.uk:80/Bandolier/band12/b12–2.html
11 http://136.159.166.5/29_Jun_1995.htm

2

Getting wired

Box 2.1 Chapter objectives

- Explain what the Internet is.

- Introduce some of the key Internet services such as e-mail and the World Wide Web (WWW).

- Provide a checklist of items required for Internet access.

- Detail the services and prices of the leading Internet service providers in the UK.

- Provide typical costing for Internet connectivity.

INTRODUCTION

Having seen that the Internet can provide you with relevant, timely, and unique information resources, it is necessary to set about the task of getting connected. Before doing this, however, it is important to have some understanding of what the Internet actually is.

What is the Internet?

Put simply, the Internet is a network of computer networks that spans the globe. In terms of size, a survey conducted in January 1996 calculated that the Internet consists of around 95 000 autonomous computer networks, providing connectivity in over 130 countries.[1]

What makes the Internet so remarkable is the fact that all these computers, on all these separate networks, can all communicate with each other. This situation has been made possible by the fact that they all speak the same language. For the more technically minded, all computers connected to the Internet use the same protocols, namely TCP/IP (transmission control protocol/Internet protocol).

This agreed protocol also means that the Internet is not platform-dependent. Though it may be slightly more complicated to get an Amiga or an Atari computer connected – in the sense that there is less Internet software available for such platforms – once a version of TCP/IP has been installed, these computers will be able to carry out the same Internet functions as an Apple Macintosh, an IBM-compatible computer, or indeed a UNIX-based system.

For the beginner, one of the key things to remember is that there is no central 'Internet computer'. For example, when you require a document published by the National Institutes of Health (NIH) you obtain it directly from a computer (known as a server) located within the NIH. Similarly, to see this week's edition of the *Weekly Epidemiological Report*, produced by the World Health Organization (WHO), the WHO server in Geneva is accessed.

If, however, you are going to access the Internet through the telephone network, the prospect of reading and fetching files from around the world raises the spectre of high telephone bills. Though access costs are discussed more fully below, it should be stressed that once you connect to your Internet provider – ideally via a local telephone number – there are no further costs relating to distance. In other words, for a UK user it costs no more to fetch a file from a server in Australia than it does to obtain it from a server in London. And strange as it may seem, if the Australian server is quiet (perhaps you are accessing it when local users are asleep), and the London server busy, you may actually get information delivered more quickly – and, therefore, more cheaply – from the site on the other side of the world.

History of the Internet

Originally devised in the 1960s as a project to ensure that military personnel could continue to communicate with each other in the event of war, the Internet has evolved into a network that interconnects government and education, and, more recently, business and commerce.

To meet the original objective, the network was built on the premise that if one part of the network failed – in cold war terms a city may be knocked out by a nuclear strike – then the message (or file) would be routed via another part. This re-routing would continue until the message reached the intended recipient.

Though, today, networks are more likely to be brought down by workmen digging up cables, the same architecture is still in place. If you look at the top part of any e-mail message you will see the route that the mail has taken. Every server that forwards the mail 'stamps' it with the server name, and the date and time.

The explosion of interest in the Internet is, however, a relatively recent phenomenon. In 1981, the Internet Society counted 500 host computers on the Internet. Ten years later, this figure had increased to 100 000. By 1996, this number had soared to more than 9 million.[2,3]

This massive upturn in the popularity of the Internet was bought about by the development of the World Wide Web and more specifically the release, in December 1993, of *Mosaic*, the first graphical World Wide Web browser.

Moreover, this explosion of interest in, and development of, the Internet shows no sign of abating. The Internet Society has calculated that a new network joins the Internet every 30 minutes.[4] More spectacularly, it appears that the total number of Web sites is doubling every five months.[5] The number of individual people who can now access the Internet is estimated to be around 30 million, and current projections suggest that if demand continued to increase at the present rate, every person on the planet could be connected by 2003.[6]

SOME KEY SERVICES

This section introduces you to the primary Internet tools and services. This however is not an exhaustive list. Facilities such as PING – through which you can check whether or not another computer on the network is available – or the more mysterious-sounding finger, will not be discussed. If you require information on these, and other advanced Internet tools, see the *Electronic Frontiers Foundation (Extended) Guide to the Internet* at:

http://www.ast.cam.ac.uk/documents/Internet

E-mail

The desire to communicate electronically with colleagues and friends is still the principal reason why people seek Internet connectivity. In its simplest form e-mail (electronic mail) can be used to send messages consisting of nothing other than text from one location to another. Beyond this, it can be used to send binary files such as word-processed documents, or act as an information retrieval tool.

The popularity of e-mail can be put down to the following factors: it is cheap, easy to use, quick, and very efficient. Chapter 6 amplifies these points, and demonstrates why e-mail has become an indispensable tool for all Internet users.

World Wide Web – WWW

The development of the World Wide Web has provided the Internet with a multimedia interface. Using a mark-up language known as HTML, Web documents (called pages) can include text, graphics, moving images and sound. To 'read' a Web page you need a Web browser, such as Mosaic, Netscape, or Internet Explorer. Appendix B contains details of how to use *Netscape*.

One of the attractions of the Web is the way in which related documents are seamlessly linked. As you scroll through a Web page, various words and phrases are highlighted or underlined, indicating that these are hypertext links (Fig. 2.1). Mouse-clicking on one of these links sends a command to your Web browser to access this related resource. The page that is subsequently displayed may reside within the same file as the original document, in a different file on the same server, or in a different file on a different server anywhere in the world.

Because the Web browser is recognised as the 'killer application', relatively little attention is now paid to its immediate predecessor, Gopher. Gopher provided the first menu-

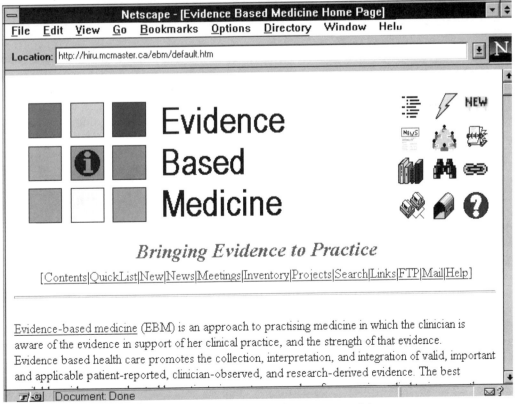

Fig. 2.1 World Wide Web page: underlined words and the graphics are hypertext links

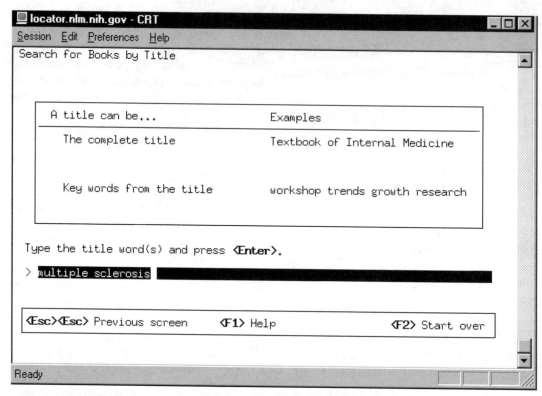

Fig. 2.2   Searching the NLM book catalogue via Telnet

driven, text-based interface to the Internet. However, as Gopher resources can be accessed through your Web browser, they will not be dealt with separately in this book.

File transfer protocol

File transfer protocol (FTP) is the set of rules that govern how files on the Internet are moved from one location to another. For further information about FTP see 'Finding and FTPing software' below.

Telnet

Telnet is a service that enables you to connect to remote computers on the Internet, and use them in the same way as you would if you were sitting in front of them. Unlike the Web, however, Telnet does not support a graphical interface (Figs 2.2, 2.3). The task of having to remember obscure key-stroke commands, such as pressing the Ctrl and x keys simulta-

neously to end a Telnet session, can be a difficult and frustrating experience after the elegance and simplicity of the Web.

Because of these perceived difficulties, owners of Telnet sites are beginning to make their services available via the Web. However, until this process is complete, if you wish to access valuable resources such as Uncover[7] – the contents page service developed by Blackwells – or the book catalogue of National Library of Medicine (NLM)[8], then Telnet is your only option.

Usenet News

Usenet News – or network news as it is sometimes referred to – is the Internet equivalent of a bulletin board system. Through this Internet service, it is possible to engage in a subject-specific *group* discussion with other Internet users. Many of these groups are highly specialised, as is testified by the fact that there are approximately 15 000 different newsgroups.

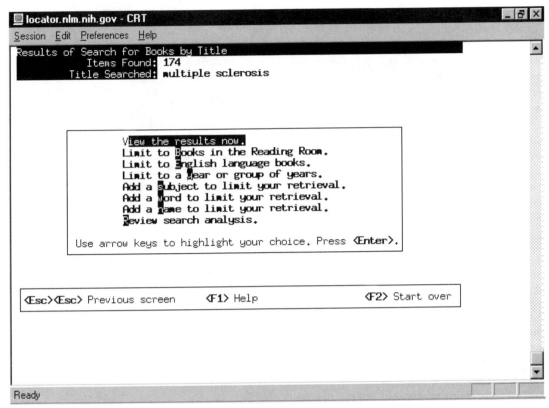

Fig. 2.3   Results of a the search of the NLM book catalogue

Chapter 6 looks in more detail at this subject, and highlights those newsgroups of most interest to health professionals.

GETTING CONNECTED

Note   The purpose of this section is to give practical advice on how you can get your computer connected to the Internet. In doing this, it is assumed that the connection will be made via a dial-up commercial Internet provider. If you already have access to the Internet via JANET, or some other institutional network, and you do not wish to have a connection at home, some of the following discussion may not be relevant.

Though a glance along the shelves of any computer bookstore may convince you otherwise, getting connected to the Internet is *not* difficult. Box 2.2 identifies the sum total of items needed for Internet connectivity. Further details of these components are discussed below.

The computer

It is possible to hook up almost any computer, with any specification, to the Internet. However, if you want to enjoy the benefits of a graphical environment (Windows or Apple Macintosh), then the minimum *acceptable* configuration is a computer with a 486 processor that has at least 4 MB (megabytes) of RAM (random access memory).

Box 2.2   Necessary components for Internet connectivity

- A computer
- A modem
- A telephone line
- An account with an Internet provider
- A copy of TCP/IP communications software
- Some Internet application software

Though it is technically possible to run Windows software on a 386PC, in terms of connecting to the Internet, I would not recommend it. The loading of image-rich Web pages would be painfully slow, and multitasking on such a machine – receiving mail in one window for example, whilst browsing the Web in another – would be all but impossible.

As with all computer programs, the more power you have, in terms of processor size, clock speed and RAM, the better the applications perform. In this sense at least, the Internet is no different. Appendix C gives details on how you can 'tweak' your computer to optimise its performance for Internet-specific tasks.

Choosing your modem

Modems are the clever bits of equipment that connect a computer to a data-transmission line; in the case of connecting to the Internet this is a telephone line. How they actually work is beyond the scope of this book. What *is* important is to purchase a modem that will perform the task of getting data from the Internet to your computer quickly and efficiently. Box 2.3 highlights the factors you need to consider to realise this objective.

As a rule of thumb, there should be no need to learn the intricacies of the AT command language – a strange language only modems really understand – nor to alter any of the DIP switches. The modem factory-settings should be correct for Internet connectivity.

CHOOSING AN INTERNET PROVIDER

An Internet provider is a company that has a permanent connection to the Internet and who, for a fee, will let you use this route to access the Internet. Once connected to your provider, via a telephone line, you are effectively connected to the Internet. You will have your own unique Internet address, be able to transfer files directly to your hard disk, and access such facilities as the World Wide Web, Gopher, and e-mail. When you have finished browsing the Web or sending your mail, you

---

Box 2.3   Choosing a modem: factors to consider

- Modem speeds are measured in bits per second (bps). Ensure that the one you buy can transmit and receive data *at least* as fast as that provided by your Internet provider. Most providers now support the V34 standard, which equates to 28 800 bps. Communicating at the maximum possible speed ensures that your telephone bills are kept to a minimum.

- Ensure that the modem supports error correction and data compression.

- Purchase a shielded modem cable. Fast modems interface with the computer using a process called hard handshaking that allows your computer to sense how data is flowing to and from your modem. Without a shielded cable this process cannot occur, and consequently you will suffer 'overruns'. When this occurs the data you have requested has to be re-transmitted, and this results in longer on-line times.

- Ask your Internet provider to recommend a modem. If you do experience problems establishing a connection, the fewer variables in the equation the better. Buying a modem that your provider knows has not caused any problems to other users removes one such variable.

---

log off. As your provider remains connected all the time, any mail sent to you when you are not connected, is held by your provider and delivered to you when you next log on.

Choosing which Internet provider to sign up with is not so straightforward. At the time of writing, there are over 120 companies in the UK offering Internet connectivity. To help select the provider that can best address your needs, consider the points in Box 2.4.

The key Internet providers in the UK

With many things to consider, and numerous companies offering connectivity, selecting the right Internet provider can be a difficult and time consuming process. To assist you in this task, Tables 2.1 to 2.6 compare the services and prices of the leading Internet providers in the UK. Figures 2.4 to 2.9 show their associated Home Pages.

Box 2.4 What to look for from an Internet provider

- Does the Internet provider have a *local* point of presence (PoP)? To ensure that your telephone bill does not resemble your telephone number, it is crucial that you can dial your provider via a local telephone number.

- Costs. Ensure that the costs of your Internet provider are clearly defined. Is there a registration fee, or are costs related to how much mail you send or how long you spend connected?

- What is the user: modem ratio? Industry experts believe that the minimum acceptable ratio is 30 users per modem. Thus, if your Internet provider boasts of having 30 000 subscribers it should have 1000 modems so that 1000 subscribers can be connected at any one time. If this ratio is exceeded, expect to experience the 'busy' dialling tone.

- Getting started. Will the Internet provider supply you with a suite of Internet-ready programs that can be installed with ease?

- Support. If you think that you may need quite a lot of help to get started, choose an Internet provider that can genuinely offer this service. This can be tested quite simply by telephoning the help line. If you succeed in getting through to their help desk (and not just their switchboard) then they probably have enough staff to assist. If the help desk is permanently engaged, then try another provider.

Note All data in the Tables is subject to change. This data was validated in March 1996.

Selection criteria

With one exception, CompuServe, only those companies who are members of London Internet Exchange (LINX) *and* meet the additional criteria cited below, are included in this list of key providers.

Membership to LINX is restricted to Internet service providers (ISPs) who have their own international connectivity, and thus are independent of any other provider. Companies such as the BBC Networking Club, Cityscape, and Direct Connection are excluded, as their networks belong to another provider, namely PIPEX, Demon and EuNet.

In addition to being an independent ISP, I deemed that key providers must also:

- aim their service at the home user (this principle excludes almost half of the 16 members of LINX);
- have a minimum of 8 PoPs – most have many more;
- offer full Internet access – not just e-mail;
- provide new subscribers with 'getting started' software for PC and Apple Macintosh market.

CompuServe is included here because it is the biggest on-line service provider in Europe, with over 200 000 individual subscribers.

For information on other Internet providers, I recommend you visit your local newsagent and scan through some of the current Internet magazines (Appendix A). Once you have a working Internet connection, a complete listing of UK providers and the services they offer can be found at:

http://www.limitless.co.uk/inetuk

DIALLING INTO THE INTERNET

To be able to connect to the Internet through your provider, you must use communications software that supports the Internet protocols, TCP/IP. Programs such as *Windows Terminal* or *Datatalk*, do *not* support this protocol and, therefore, cannot be used.

In addition to acquiring TCP/IP, you will need a copy of either SLIP or PPP software. These are 'drivers' that enable TCP/IP to work over serial lines, such as the telephone network.

As your Internet provider will supply you with copies of the required software and drivers, plus additional software to help you install and configure these, further explanation of TCP/IP, SLIP and PPP is unnecessary. It is mentioned here is simply to reinforce the fact that you need these additional items before you can connect to the Internet.

Table 2.1   The Cable Online service

Provider	Joining fee	Monthly fee	PoPs in UK	User: modem ratio	Maximum connect speed
Cable Online	£20.00	£14.95	15	Not available (see below)	All PoPs 28.8 kbps

Other costs	None

Comments	• Membership comes complete with the *Netscape* World Wide Web browser, *Eudora Light* e-mail client, and a getting started tutorial disk.
	• For an additional £19.95, Cable Online offers users an optional software package called *CyberPatrol* that automatically blocks access to Internet sites known to offer sensitive or offensive material. This list of sites is updated every 7 days, making it extremely unlikely that you, your colleagues or your children will stumble across anything that might offend.
	• Though Cable Online do not publish figures relating to the user:modem ratio, they publicly guarantee that subscribers will only experience the engaged tone one time in a hundred.[9]

Contact	**Tel: 0800 506 506** **http://www.cableol.net/**

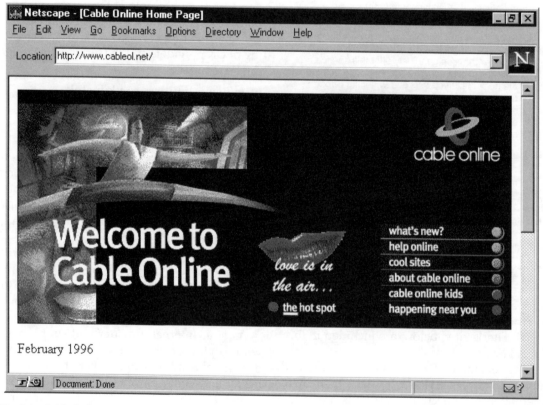

Fig. 2.4   Cable Online Home Page

Table 2.2   The CompuServe service

Provider	Joining fee	Monthly fee	PoPs in UK	User: modem ratio	Maximum connect speed
CompuServe *Standard*	Free	£6.50	8	Not available	28.8 kbps (London, B'ham and Manchester) 14.4 kbps at other nodes
CompuServe *Value Plus*	Free	£16.95			

Other costs   For the *Standard* service you are entitled to 5 hours free connect time each month. Every hour thereafter costs £1.95. In the *Value Plus* option you are given up to 20 hours free connect time every month, with additional connect time being charged at £1.50 hour. CompuServe can also be accessed via the Mercury 5000 and the GNS DialPlus networks. Though these provide additional local connectivity, they also incur an additional surcharge.

Comments   • CompuServe is one of the few companies that bases its charges on usage. If you consider 5 hours Internet connection time per month to be sufficient, then the *Standard* account is by far the cheapest way to get connected to the Internet. If you routinely exceed this 5-hour ration, then the *Value Plus* plan, or another provider may be more cost effective.

   • As CompuServe also have PoPs throughout Europe and America, this service may appeal to the travelling Internet user.

Contact   **Tel: 0800 289378**
   http://www.compuserve.com/

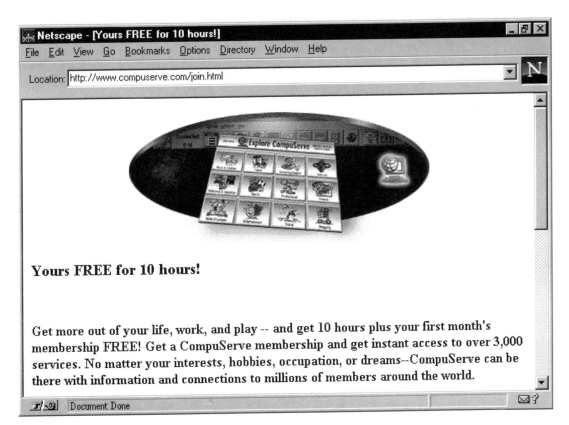

Fig. 2.5   *CompuServe Home Page*

Table 2.3   The Demon Internet service

Provider	Joining fee	Monthly fee	PoPs in UK	User: modem ratio	Maximum connect speed
Demon	£12.50	£10.00	114	Not available (see below)	All PoPs 28.8 kbps

Other costs   None

Comments

- Demon is the only company that offers local call access to the *whole* of the UK, including the Channel Islands and the Isle of Man.
- Large subscriber base (around 45 000) with very active Demon-specific newsgroups.
- Because the user base is so large, and usage patterns disparate, Demon do not consider the user:modem ratio to be a particularly meaningful way of measuring network accessibility. The official statement on this question is that 'there are sufficient modems so that the only cause of busy tones will be a failure condition or a very rare call set-up clash. It is Demon's intention to maintain as an absolute minimum a sufficient number of modems that in the peak 15 minute period 95% of callers obtain a connection within 5 attempts.'[10]
- Demon have established a large World Wide Web <u>proxy server</u>. If the Web page you seek has previously been accessed by another Demon customer, getting it from this proxy server will reduce waiting time and improve overall performance. This proxy server can <u>cache</u> up to 8 Gb of data.

Contact   **Tel: 0181 371 1234**
http://www.demon.co.uk/

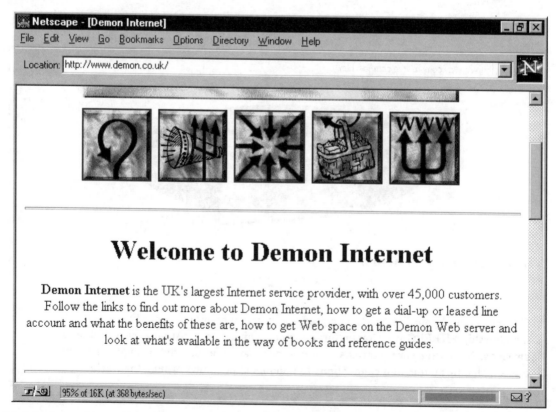

Fig. 2.6   Demon Internet Home Page

Table 2.4   The IBM Global service

Provider	Joining fee	Monthly fee	PoPs in UK	User: modem ratio	Maximum connect speed
IBM Global *Standard*	Waived for '96	£10.00	11	Not available	28.8 kbps at 3 PoPs,
IBM Global *Comprehensive*	Waived for '96	£20.00			14.4 kbps at the other 8 PoPs

Other costs   With the *Standard* account you are entitled to 3 hours free connection time in any month. Each hour thereafter costs £3.00. With the *Comprehensive* plan you are entitled to 30 hours free connection time in any month. Each hour thereafter costs £3.00.

Comments
- With 570 access numbers across the world it will appeal to the travelling Internet user.
- A recognised name. Better the devil you know?

Contact   **Tel: 0800 963949**
http://www.ibm.net/

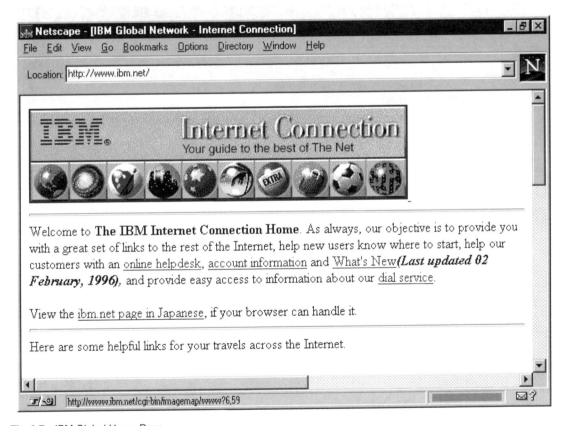

Fig. 2.7   IBM Global Home Page

Table 2.5   The Netkonect service

Provider	Joining fee	Monthly fee	PoPs in UK	User: modem ratio	Maximum connect speed
Netkonect	£0.00	£10.00	60	25:1	All PoPs 28.8 kbps

Other costs   None

Comments
- Netkonect *guarantee* a maximum user: modem ratio of 25:1
- If you are prepared to pay a year's subscription in advance, then the cost per month drops to £8.50. This makes it one of the cheapest Internet providers in the UK.
- A new users starting page that contains links to Web search engines and popular Web sites.
- Provide a FTP server that contains popular and useful software.

Contact   **Tel: 01420 542777**
http://www.netkonect.net/

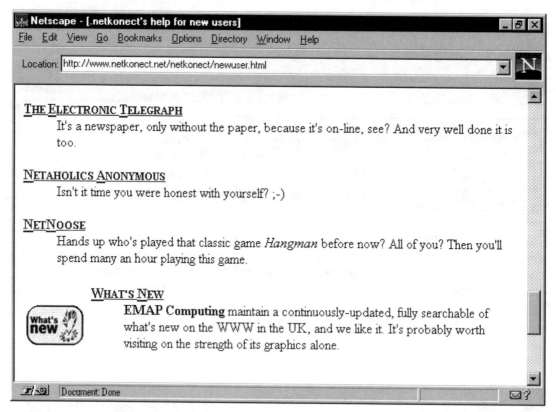

Fig. 2.8   Netkonect New Users Home Page

Table 2.6 The Unipalm PIPEX service

Provider	Joining fee	Monthly fee	PoPs in UK	User: modem ratio	Maximum connect speed
Unipalm PIPEX	£50.00 (with software) £10.00 (no software)	£15.00 £15.00	53	Not available	All PoPs 28.8 kbps

Other costs	None
Comments	• 53 PoPs in the UK means that approximately 90% of the UK is covered by a local PoP.
	• PIPEX provide a sophisticated <u>plug and play</u> package that simplifies the task of getting your computer 'Internet ready'.
	• All subscribers are given 0.5 MB of space on the PIPEX World Wide Web server. This means than *every* user can have a presence on the Web. To ensure that subscribers can take advantage of this service, a variety of HTML guides and tutorials are also available from PIPEX.
Contact	**Tel: 0500 474739** **http://www.unipalm.pipex.com/dial/**

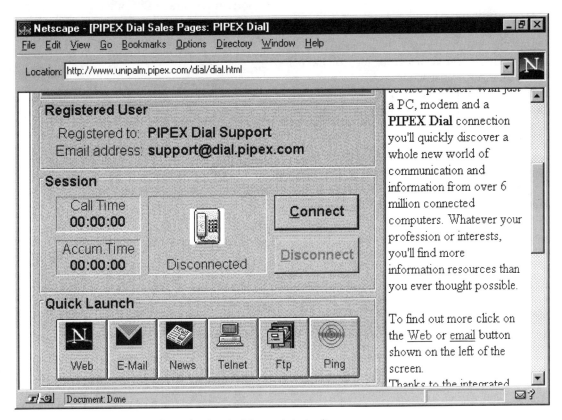

Fig. 2.9 Uniaplm PIPEX Home Page showing the 'plug and play' software

A note for Windows 95, System 7.5 and OS/2 users

If your computer is running any of the above operating systems, it will have been shipped as 'Internet ready'. Apple's System 7.5 comes with MacTCP, whilst both the Windows95 and OS/2 products include TCP/IP software. For details on how to configure Windows95 for Internet access see Appendix D.

INTERNET SOFTWARE

The final thing you need before you can start exploring the wonders of the Internet, is some application software. For example, to send and receive e-mail, you need an e-mail program; to view pages on the World Wide Web you need a Web browser.

Most applications you use on the Internet are based on the client-server model. In very simple terms this means that you have a copy of the software on your computer (the client) that processes requests to other computers (servers) on the Internet. For the Internet user, the advantages of this model are twofold; first, all the processing power of your computer can be harnessed and exploited, and secondly, you get to use the Internet via a graphical interface.

As mentioned earlier, your Internet provider should supply you with a suite of applications to get you started. However, as soon as you wish to add to, or change the software you use, then the resources of the Internet are at your fingertips. One of the things you will not find in short supply on the Internet is software!

To move files (in this case software) from a server on the Internet to your computer, you use the Internet protocol, FTP.

Finding and FTPing software

The techniques discussed in Chapter 3 for finding medical information can also be used to identify where a particular computer program can be found on the Internet. For example, to acquire a new e-mail client you can visit the Yahoo index[11] and follow the hypertext links from 'Computers and Internet' to 'Software', and through to 'Electronic-Mail'. At this juncture, you will find yourself presented with a choice of around 20 different mail programs.

Once you have identified which piece of software you require, it can be FTPd to your computer by simply mouse-clicking on the file name. The Web browser will immediately realise that the file cannot be viewed and suggest that it should be saved to disk. Depending on which browser you are running, you may see a 'saving' dialogue box that indicates how much of the file has been transferred, and approximately how long it will take to complete this task (Fig. 2.10).

Moving files in this way is often referred to as 'anonymous FTP'. The reason for this is that you log on to the server under the name 'anonymous' and use your e-mail address as your password. (If you FTP through your Web browser and have entered your e-mail address in the 'Preferences Settings', you will never be prompted for this information (Appendix B)).

An alternative approach to finding software is to visit a suitably large archive, and browse. In the UK, the main repository of software is held on a server at the Imperial College in London. To use this resource, point your Web browser at:

http://src.doc.ic.ac.uk/

In common with other FTP sites, files at Imperial are arranged hierarchically. Thus, software for the IBM-compatible PC, or the Apple Mac can be found under the folders 'ibmpc' and 'mac' respectively. Within each folder further sub-divisions are introduced to facilitate retrieval (Fig. 2.11).

If you know the name of the file you are looking for, the search engine at Imperial can be used to identify its precise location. If required, this tool can be instructed to search not only the local server (i.e. Imperial), but all the FTP sites in the world. Beware though, you may have to wait some considerable time for this.

One other invaluable UK FTP site is the University of Lancaster's Higher Education National Software Archive (HENSA).[12] Here, software can be searched for by platform, by

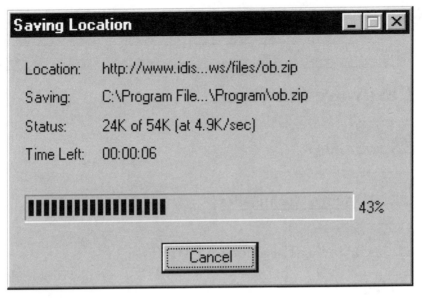

Fig. 2.10 Saving a file using *Netscape*

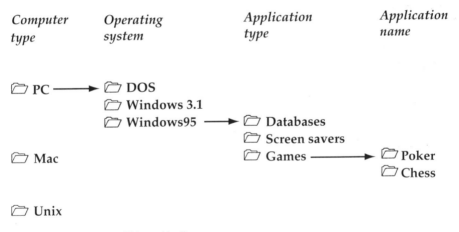

Fig. 2.11 FTP sites: files are arranged hierarchically

keyword or, if you are looking for a popular piece of software, simply by consulting the 'top 50' most referenced packages (Figs 2.12, 2.13).

This site can be reached by pointing your Web browser at:

http://micros.hensa.ac.uk

If you are accessing the HENSA archive from a non-academic <u>domain name</u> – that is, your Internet address does not include **.ac.** –

then access to this site is prohibited between 8.00 a.m. and 8.00 p.m. GMT.

Installing FTPd software

To speed up data transfer, most software applications are delivered to your computer in a compressed format. This either takes the form of a self-extracting archive, or a packed file. In the former case, you simply need to run the program to create all the necessary files

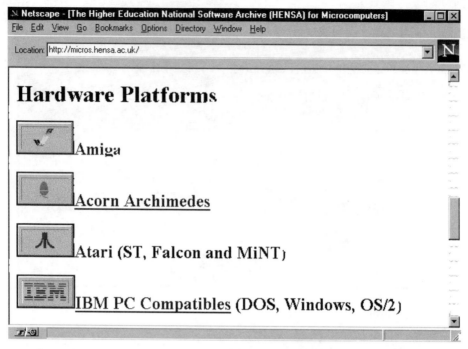

Fig. 2.12 The HENSA archive: finding software compatible with your operating system

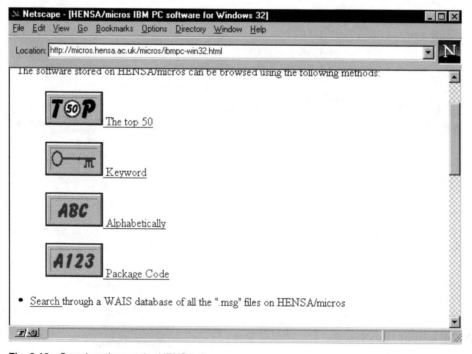

Fig. 2.13 Search options at the HENSA site

and directories. If the file has been packed, you need to unpack it. Depending upon your operating platform, decompression utilities can be FTPd from the following sites:

- IBMPC:
  ftp://ftp.pkware.com/pub/pkware

- Apple Macintosh:
  http://pubweb.nexor.co.uk/public/mac/ archive/welcome.html

Once unpacked, instructions on how to install the software will be found in a 'readme' file.

Shareware and freeware

Newcomers to the Internet are often amazed at how easy it is to FTP software, and do so without having to quote credit card details, or an official purchase order number. Most software on the Internet is classified as shareware, which normally means that you are entitled to use it and evaluate it for a period of around 30 days. After this time, if you wish to continue using the software you are obliged to register your copy, and pay a fairly nominal licence fee.

Registration not only legitimises your use of the software, but may also entitle you to some additional documentation or e-mail support. The cost of some of the more popular Internet shareware is shown in Table 2.7.

Other useful utilities

Your Web browser can be called upon to carry out many more functions than simply displaying World Wide Web pages. It can FTP as competently as a specific FTP program. It can display bitmap (<u>bmp</u>) and JPEG (<u>jpg</u>) images and, if you have a <u>sound card</u> in your computer, play audio clips. Developments in recent months have also enabled some browsers, such as Netscape and the Microsoft Explorer, to compose, send and, if you have a <u>POP3</u> mail account, receive electronic mail.

Web browsers cannot, however, run Telnet sessions or play video clips. To find clients that can carry out these tasks, visit the HENSA FTP site discussed above, and undertake a search using the keywords 'Telnet' 'MPEG' and '<u>Quicktime</u>'. Appendix B details how these applications can be launched through the Netscape browser to create a seamless interface.

One other piece of software worth acquiring is a <u>virus</u> checker. Though the hype about viruses on the Internet has been overplayed, they do exist and should be taken seriously. The recently discovered 'winword.concept' virus – which hides itself as a macro in a Microsoft *Word* template document – demonstrates the skill and ingenuity of the people who create these viruses. Chapter 6 gives details on e-mail viruses.

To negate this threat, all Internet users should invest in anti-virus software. Before purchasing this, check with the supplier that the software can check *compressed* files for viruses. If a virus is within a piece of software, simply 'unpacking' it may infect your computer.

Table 2.7 Software registration fees: some typical examples

Software	Function	Cost
Trumpet Winsock	TCP/IP & SLIP/PPP communications software	US$25.00 (£16.50)
MacTCP	TCP/IP communications software for the Mac	US$42.00 (£27.50)
Netscape	World Wide Web browser	US$39.00 (£24.00)
Pegasus	Windows e-mail program	Freeware

Table 2.8 Getting connected: costs

Description	Average cost
Modem (one-off cost)	£160.00
Client software (one-off cost)	£50.00
Internet provider membership fee (one-off cost)	£12.00
Annual subscription to your Internet provider	£120.00
Total cost for year 1 (excluding VAT)	£342.00

COSTS

Perhaps the most surprising thing about the Internet is how little it all costs. Leaving aside telephone charges for the moment, the cost of a year's access to the Internet is likely to be around £120.00. When you consider that a personal subscription to a journal such as the *Lancet* is a similar sum you begin to appreciate what good value the Internet is.[13] Table 2.8 details *all* the initial charges you are likely to incur.

Though telephone costs are the great variable in the cost equation, they are the one feature over which you have total control. To help keep them to an affordable level, I suggest you adhere to the points in Box 2.5.

CONCLUSION

This chapter has demonstrated that connecting your computer to the Internet is a relatively straightforward operation, and one that does not entail huge costs. Once connectivity has been achieved, the resources of the world are just a mouse-click away.

Box 2.5 Minimising your telephone costs

- Always dial your local point of presence.
- Always connect at the fastest possible modem speed.
- If you can, defer access until off-peak telephone rates apply.
- Plan what you want to do on the Internet *before* you log on, and try to stick to this. Though browsing on the Internet is highly enjoyable (and addictive), be conscious of how much this costs and calculate whether the information you glean is worth the expense.
- Keep FTPing of computer programs to a minimum. Programs, by their very nature, tend to be large and therefore relatively expensive to FTP.
- When you have to FTP a computer program (or any large file), try to do this at a time when the Internet is less busy. For UK users this means FTPing in the mornings, before the US users have woken up and logged on.
- Configure your Web browser so that graphics are *not* displayed. This will result in Web pages being displayed more quickly, thereby enabling a faster and cheaper Internet session (Appendix B).
- Compose and read e-mail off-line.
- Compose and read Usenet News off-line.
- Use this book as your off-line reference guide.

REFERENCES AND NOTES

1 http://www.nw.com/
2 ftp://ftp.isoc.org/isoc/charts/network-gifs/overall.gif
3 http://www.nw.com/
4 ftp://ftp.isoc.org/isoc/charts/history-gifs/timeline.gif
5 Gray M .net Genesis. Article at:
   http://www.netgen.com/infoarea/growth.html
6 Anon. .Net: the Internet Magazine 1995 1 (2):15
7 telnet://database.carl.org/
8 telnet://locator@locator.nlm.nih.gov/

9 Cable Online What is the Internet? Publicity brochure 1996
10 http://www.demon.co.uk/dil/connect/popfaq.html
11 http://www.yahoo.com/
12 HENSA /micros is funded by JISC for the UK Higher Education Community.
13 According to *Dawson's Guide to International Journals and Periodicals* 1995 (91st edn.), the price of the *Lancet* is £145.00.

3

Finding what you want

Box 3.1	Chapter objectives

- Introduce you to the primary search tools now available on the Internet.
- Describe, compare and assess these tools.
- Demonstrate, with practical examples, how these tools can be used to find resources to answer specific medical queries.

INTRODUCTION

Having succeeded in getting your computer hooked up to the Internet, almost certainly your first question will be, 'How do I find information relevant to my needs?' Answering that question is the purpose of this chapter.

At the start, it should be pointed out that there is no right or wrong way to search the Internet. Undoubtedly, some methods may be more time-consuming than others, but in the end you must choose the method that best suits you. As you come to explore the Internet you will soon appreciate why your Web browser is so named. In my trawls of the Internet I have often come across extremely useful resources simply by browsing and following a series of hypertext links.

Essentially you can search for information in the following ways:

- by using a **free-text** search engine to interrogate a database of Internet resources;
- by browsing/searching through **subject-arranged** resource lists;
- by browsing/searching through **evaluated** sources of information.

This chapter looks in detail at each of these and highlights the strengths and weaknesses of each method. Throughout, the discussion is punctuated with examples of search questions and descriptions of what was found. Each section concludes with a 'worked example' demonstrating how a specific medical query was answered. These can subsequently be used as templates for any information search you may wish to undertake.

FREE-TEXT SEARCHING

Given its size, one of the more remarkable features of the Internet is the fact that it is possible to search for information by key-words. The user, looking for information on say, 'gene therapy', simply enters this term in a search query-box, and within a matter of seconds a list of Internet sites that discuss this topic is displayed.

This function has been made possible by the development of computer programs known as robots. (Occasionally, you may see these referred to as 'spiders', 'worms' or 'know-bots'.) In very simple terms, a robot wanders around the Internet gathering details of what is available.[1] Retrieved data is added to a database that can subsequently be searched. Figure 3.1 shows how users interrogate such a database via a typical graphical query-form.

At present, there are at least a dozen robot-generated Internet databases available for searching. Unfortunately, as these databases are constructed in different ways, a search undertaken on one and then repeated on

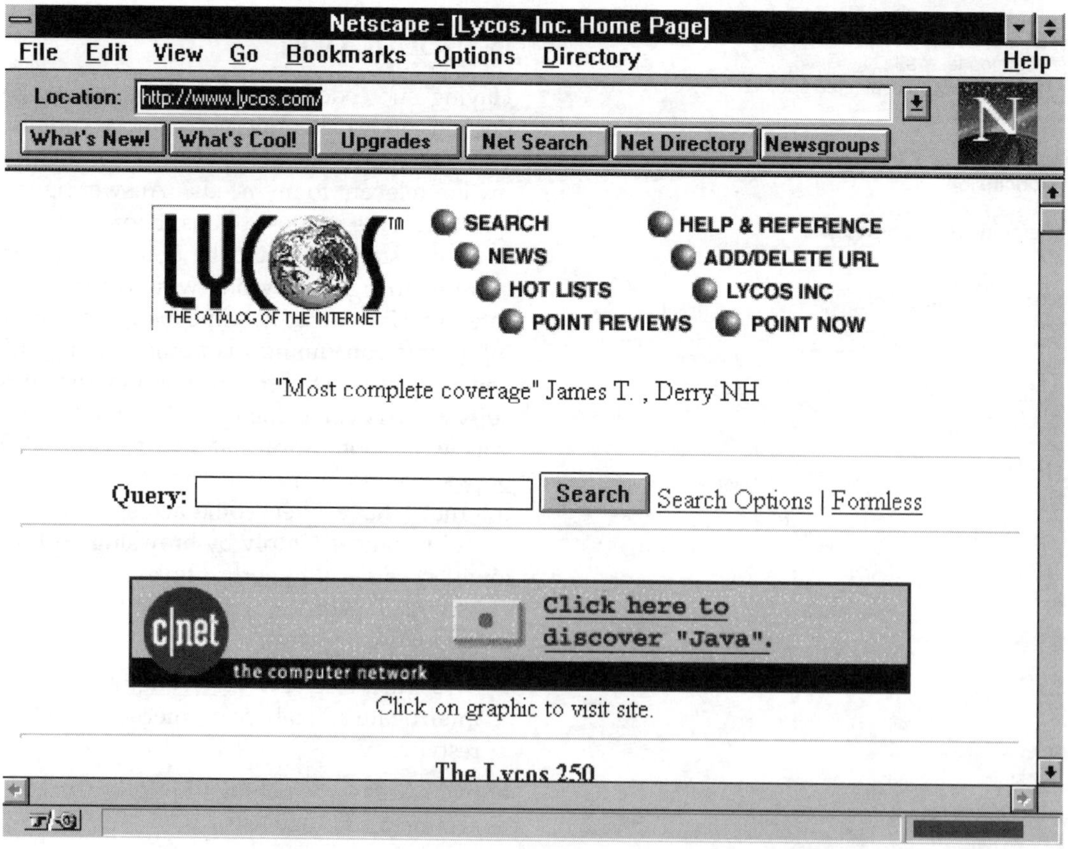

Fig. 3.1 Typical query-form search interface

another, may produce widely contrasting results. The reasons for this are many, but the two major factors are:

- each database proprietor decides *which* Internet resources are to be included and which are to be excluded (thus some databases include FTP and Gopher resources, whereas others only index world wide web pages);

- each database proprietor decides *how* these resources are indexed (some databases only index the first 100 or so words from a document, whereas others will index every single word from every single page).

Consequently, if you are to search the Internet in a thorough and effective fashion, you need to be aware of a range of Internet indexes, and cognisant with the construction of each database. With these objectives in mind, the two biggest and most popular databases, Lycos and Open Text, are discussed below.

Lycos

http://www.lycos.com/

Without doubt, 'the catalogue of the Internet' is the biggest single index to the Internet. In February 1996, Lycos claimed to have indexed some 91% of the Internet which then amounted to over 19 million URLs. Included in this database are World Wide Web documents, FTP archives, Gopher menus, and individual binary files, such as video files and images.

How is Lycos constructed?

When the Lycos robot finds an Internet resource, it records and subsequently indexes the URL, data from the title and header fields,[2] the 100 'most statistically salient words',[3] and the first 20 lines of the document. Data that resides beyond these boundaries are not included and thus cannot be searched for.

Searching Lycos

To search the Lycos database you enter your term(s) in the query-box and press the *Search* button. When the search has been executed, the results are displayed in a ranked order, with the most relevant document at the top of the list. The ranking of sites is based on the popularity of the document, which is calculated by looking at the total number of *other* sites that contain links to that page. A search on 'gulf war syndrome' for example, will find all pages in the Lycos database that contain these three words. At the *top* of the list however, will be the site that other Internet documents reference most frequently. The premise is that the more a document is referenced by other Web pages, the more useful it will be.

The Lycos search engine also supports the option of finding just some of the terms in your search query. The benefits of this may not be immediately obvious, but in medicine, where many terms have both an English and American spelling, not to mention Greek or Latin roots, this is a most useful function. Asking Lycos to match just two of the terms in a search on 'community pediatrics paediatrics' should ensure that resources on this topic are not inadvertently overlooked.

On the downside however, you cannot ask Lycos to find terms that are adjacent to each other, nor can you weight a term to give it more importance. More frustratingly, because Lycos adopts an in-depth-first rather than a breadth-first approach, some searches find numerous references to the same resource. For example, a search for the 'social security manual' will not just guide you to the US Social *Service Administration* Home Page, but to all the specific sections associated with this document. For the user, this means scanning through many hits in a search for the most appropriate one.

Open Text

http://www.opentext.com/

With a database consisting of more than 16 million Internet sites and 27 million hypertext links, 'the fastest, most powerful search tool on the Internet' is the second largest index to the Internet. The database currently consists of World Wide Web documents and Gopher-based resources.

How is Open Text constructed?

Like Lycos, Open Text has a robot prowling the Internet looking for new sites to index. What distinguishes Open Text from Lycos, however, is that once a new Internet resource has been retrieved, *every single word* in that new document is added to the Open Text database and indexed.

Searching Open Text

The decision to index every word from every identified resource has inevitably led to the creation of a huge database. (In February 1996 this database consisted of some 2.5 billion words.) However, because the Open Text designers have developed a very powerful search engine, the problems normally associated with full-text databases – high recall and low precision – are not encountered. Open Text offers three types of search: simple, power and weighted.

Simple search In this option, the user enters the search term(s) in the query-box and indicates – by ticking the appropriate option – whether the database should return items that match all or some of the terms. If you have entered a phrase – 'management of diabetes' for example – you can specify that the whole phrase must be matched. Open Text is the *only* search engine that lets you perform phrase searching, without recourse to specific commands or symbols.

Power search This enables the user to specify *where* in a World Wide Web page a particular term should appear. Thus, you can specify that a keyword should appear in the title section of a Web page, whereas other, less pertinent terms, can appear anywhere in the document. Power searching also supports the facility to find terms 'near' one another, or terms that are 'followed by'. For example, the search 'asthma' *near* 'treatment' will identify resources even when these terms are not adjacent to each other.

Weighted search This option allows the user to weight terms to indicate their relative importance to a search.

Once a search has been executed, Open Text displays the results in ranked order. This ranking is based on the frequency a searched word (or phrase) appears in the document.

In addition to providing hypertext links to the suggested Internet sites, the Open Text database has two other features.

- You can see where your search terms appear in the document *before* accessing the resource. Though a 5/6 line summary of all suggested locations is displayed, it is not always obvious why a particular site has been identified. Seeing where the search term actually appears on the page can help you decide whether the site is worth a visit.

- You can run another search against the database but this time using one of the identified documents as the basis of your search (Fig. 3.2). This option to 'find similar pages' works by virtue of the fact that the Open Text search engine can calculate which terms appear most frequently in any selected document and then re-run the search using this new data.

Lycos and Open Text: some comparisons

- Because of its size and its speed of response Lycos is a most valuable search tool. However, though the find-rate is high, the relevance of the suggested documents can, on occasions, be disappointingly low.

- Open Text, being a smaller database, may identify fewer documents but this is more than compensated by the powerful and flexible search engine that can be used to perform highly precise information searches.

To compare, in a more scientific way, the relative virtues of both databases, two searches

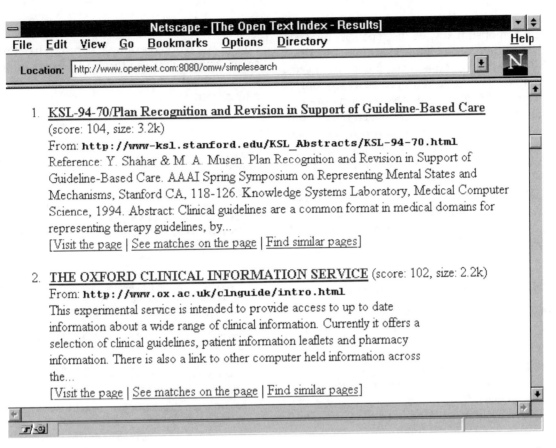

Fig. 3.2   Results from an Open Text search on 'clinical guidelines': you can always 'Visit the page', 'See matches on the page' or 'Find similar pages'

were performed. To ensure that the test was as objective as possible, both searches were carried out on the same day, both single-term and phrase searching were tested, and in both databases the default search option was used. The results of this test are shown in Table 3.1.

Results analysis

In the search on 'phacoemulsification' it was interesting to discover that though both databases identified seven sites, only *one* site was common to both. In both databases, this resource was identified as the most relevant.

Table 3.1   Comparing Lycos with Open Text: a controlled test

Database	Term search: phacoemulsification	Phrase search: adenosine deaminase deficiency
Lycos	7 hits (1 duplicate)	15 hits (5 duplicates)
Open Text	7 hits (3 duplicates)	8 hits (1 duplicate)

Note   Duplicates. On occasions a particular resource may appear in a number of different directories, or even on a number of different servers. However, because these resources have different URLs they are added to the various databases as 'original' documents. In the following test all duplicated resources are identified.

The 'adenosine deaminase deficiency' search also demonstrated wide discrepancies between the two databases. Of the 8 resources identified by Open Text, none was found by Lycos. Moreover, of the 15 retrieved by Lycos, only 1 document had all three search terms present; the other 14 documents contained only two of the three terms. Not surprisingly, these resources were perceived as the least useful.

This example demonstrates the variable results that different Internet databases can yield. Consequently, if you require an exhaustive and comprehensive search of the Internet, you must be prepared to use a range of robot-generated databases.[4]

Strengths of free-text searching

- You can undertake a very specific search and find documents that precisely match your requirements.

- The comprehensive indexing of the retrieved resources means that very few searches fail; no matter how obscure your search, there is bound to be a reference to it somewhere on the Internet.

- The databases are easy to search.

Weaknesses of free-text searching

- The non-discriminatory method of document retrieval inevitably produces a number of irrelevant leads. Though a search on the term 'stroke' will point you to useful documents such as the *Spinal Cord Injury, Stroke and Paralysis Resource Guide*,[5] the same search will also suggest resources that will help improve your putting stroke,[6] or teach you about the workings of the two-stroke motorcycle engine.[7]

- The databases cannot be browsed.

- The resources added to these databases are not evaluated in any way. So, for example, if you want to ensure that your *personal home page* can be found by one of these search engines, you can e-mail its details to the Lycos and Open Text administrators.

Using a free-text search engine

Box 3.2 is a worked example of how a free text search engine was used to find further information about some research mentioned in a newspaper.

Box 3.2 Using a free-text search engine: a worked example

A recent newspaper article made reference to a study that showed that the calcium-channel blocker, nifedipine, widely used to treat chest pain and high blood pressure, can triple the death rate amongst those taking it. Can the Internet be used to help identify this research?

Methodology
The currency of the information means that the traditional literature searching sources, <u>MEDLINE</u> and <u>Embase</u>, will not yet have indexed this reference; it should, however, be possible to find this research on the Internet. The methodology for this is detailed below.

- Load up a search engine of your choice. In this example, I selected Open Text:
http://www.opentext.com

- In the search box type in a keyword. In this example, enter 'nifedipine'.

- Open Text returns with a ranked list of possible sites. The fourth item in this list looks promising:
'HDCN–News Alerts! Hypertension, Dialysis, Clinical Nephrology
New analyses regarding the safety of calcium-channel blockers'.

- Select this link:
http://www.medtext.com/newsal.htm

- At MedText, select the option 'New analyses regarding the safety of calcium-channel blockers (Fig. 3.3).

- You are now taken to the statement from the National Heart Lung and Blood Institute (NHLBI) regarding the safety of calcium-channel blockers (Fig. 3.4). This statement provides the reader with background to the research, comment on the new analyses, the adverse effects, and conclusions. The statement is supported with references, including the new research that sparked this controversy. This citation has a hypertext link, which takes you to the abstract as published in the journal *Circulation*.

Comment
Though the number of jumps may look daunting, it in fact only took just over a minute to reach the NHLBI statement. Moreover, at the MedText site, rather than go directly to the NHLBI statement, it is possible to jump to a related press release from the American Heart Association, or an associated article in *JAMA*.

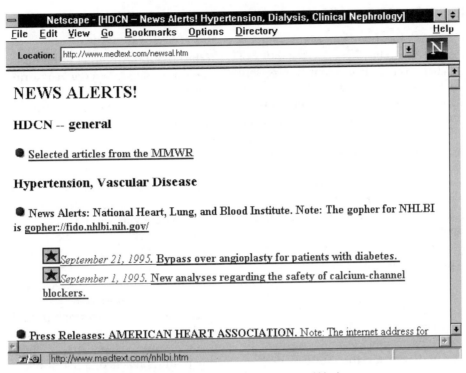

Fig. 3.3 The MedText News Alert on the safety of calcium-channel blockers

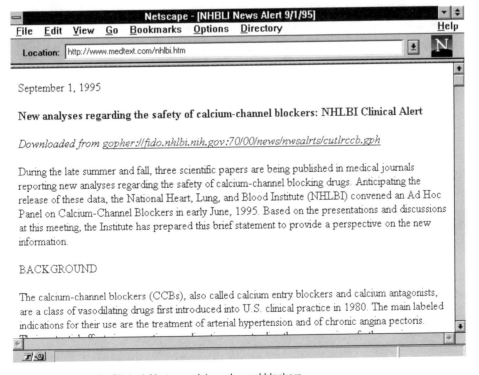

Fig. 3.4 The NHLBI Clinical Alert on calcium-channel blockers

SUBJECT CATALOGUES

In many ways, the free-text search engines described above can be likened to the index of a book. When you wish to identify precisely where in the text a specific term or concept appears, you consult the index. In contrast, when you merely require an overview of what a book is about, you examine the contents page. In this analogy, the subject catalogues are the contents pages to the Internet.

Thus, the second approach to finding medical information is to browse – or search – through a range of Internet subject catalogues. These ambitious projects attempt to arrange the resources of the Internet in the fashion of a library. To find material relating to, say, economics, one simply accesses the economics catalogue, where all material on this subject has been grouped.

For medical and health information, the most widely used subject catalogues are the Yahoo Health Pages and the World Wide Web Virtual Library, Biosciences Catalogue.

Yahoo: Health

http://www.yahoo.com/

If the size of the Internet intimidates you, then the Yahoo site is a very reassuring place to begin a search for information. Here, *all* of the resources within the Yahoo database are classified within 14 subject headings, one of which is Health.

On selecting 'Health', Yahoo begins to reveal its tight, hierarchical structure. No documents are presented to the user at this broad-concept level. Instead, Yahoo displays another menu where you select a more specific subject heading such as 'Medicine', 'Drugs' or 'Diseases'. On opting for the 'Diseases' section, Yahoo returns with yet another menu, this time inviting you to select the specific disease you are interested in.

This approach of working from the broader to the narrower concept, continues until no further sub-divisions are applicable. When this point is reached, a list of relevant sites is displayed. Figure 3.5 shows you the links

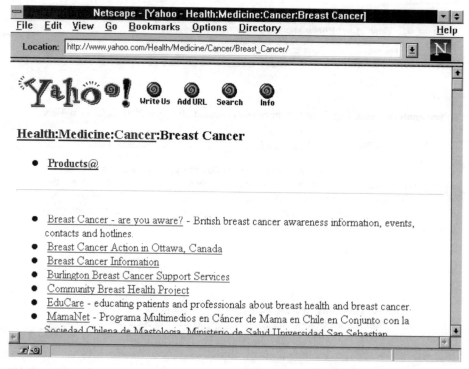

Fig. 3.5 Yahoo: Breast Cancer – the hierarchical route Health: Medicine: Cancer: Breast Cancer is displayed

available from the Breast Cancer Page, which is accessed by following the hierarchical links, 'Health', 'Medicine', 'Cancer' and 'Breast Cancer'.

If you do not know where a particular subject may fit within the classification scheme, you can search the Yahoo catalogue using its subject search engine. From the results, you can jump to the appropriate part of the subject catalogue.

By virtue of the fact that Yahoo always displays the subject heading in relation to its position in the hierarchy, you can decide whether to pursue the suggested links, or, if you feel that you have been too specific in your search, move back up the hierarchy. Continuing with the breast cancer example, mentioned above, it is possible that useful links might have been indexed under the Cancer Page. Simply by jumping back up the hierarchy, it is possible to go to the authoritative OncoLink,[8] and the National Cancer Institute,[9] both of which have numerous documents relating to breast cancer.

PC Computing described the Yahoo subject index as 'superb.'[10] Quite frankly, it is difficult to argue with this assessment.

World Wide Web Virtual Library: Medicine

http://www.w3.org/vl/
(general index)
http://www.ohsu.edu/cliniweb/wwwvl/
(medical index)
Like Yahoo, the Virtual Library arranges Internet resources hierarchically. Web sites relating to 'Medicine' are located within the Biosciences Subject Catalogue. If 'Medicine' is too general a subject heading, more specific ones such as 'Anaesthesiology', 'Epidemiology' and 'Pharmacy' are available.

From the 'Medicine' listing, one gets an idea of the wealth and diversity of medical information available on the Internet. From this single listing there are links to more than 600 health-related sites. Figure 3.6 captures a tiny part of this huge resource.

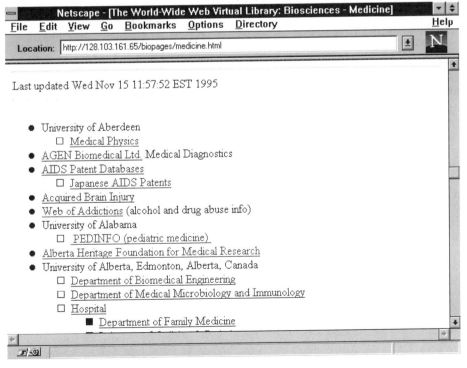

Fig. 3.6 Section of the Biosciences Virtual Library

Unlike Yahoo though, resources in the 'Medicine' subject index are not further categorised by additional indexing terms. The browseable list is alphabetically arranged by provider. Thus, Aberdeen University appears first, Yale University last. To meet the need for a subject approach, however, all the entries on any of the Biosciences pages can be searched.[11]

The Virtual Library takes the form of a 'distributed catalogue' where named individuals – or university departments – take responsibility for identifying relevant resources. The Medical Catalogue, for example, is the responsibility of Dr Richard Appleyard at Oregon Health Sciences University, whilst the Anaesthesiology Catalogue is managed by Yale University. Though this may be the only practical way to organise the workload, it results in a lack of uniformity in the way the material is presented. For example, whereas the Pharmacy Catalogue arranges the resources by country, the Epidemiology Catalogue uses a subject approach, whilst the AIDS Catalogue is just a list of resources in no recognisable order. This failure to standardise the list layout means that the user has to spend time determining how a particular part of the Virtual Library has categorised its resources.

Though the World Wide Web Virtual Library, and in particular the Biosciences subject catalogues, may not be as easy to use as Yahoo, it is included here as it is the best way of getting a flavour of *who* is publishing on the Internet, and what kind of material is currently available.

Strengths of subject catalogues

- Subject catalogues allow you to identify Internet resources from a broad subject base, thereby negating the need to identify highly specific search terms.

- Their hierarchical and browseable structure provides a logical and accessible route to the Internet and, thus, are an ideal starting point for the new user.

Weaknesses of subject catalogues

- As the creation of a subject heading requires *some* human input, the catalogues tend to be smaller and less up-to-date than their free-text equivalents.

- Relevant resources may be overlooked by the inappropriate use of subject headings. For example, the premier Internet site for disease prevention, the Centre for Diseases Control and Prevention (CDC), is only located in the Yahoo catalogue under the obscure and missable 'Government – Agencies – Executive Branch' subject heading.[12]

Using a subject catalogue

Box 3.3 is a worked example of using a subject catalogue to find information relating to midwifery.

Box 3.3   Using a subject catalogue: a worked example

A midwife, on reading that the Internet has resources that are of use to all health professionals, wants to know what is available in the general area of midwifery.

Methodology
As this is such a general enquiry, the free-text databases that search for individual Internet resources will not be of great use. Though one could search for the term 'midwifery' it is likely that potentially relevant sites would be overlooked. A resource on breast-feeding or caesarean section, for example, that may be of interest to the midwife would be missed if these sites did not include the specific word 'midwifery'. Consequently, a better approach is to use an Internet subject catalogue. The methodology and results are described below.

- Call up the Yahoo subject catalogue:
http://www.yahoo.com/
I selected this catalogue as it is the easiest one to use.

- From the 'Health' subject category follow the links to 'Nursing' and then 'Midwifery'. If you did not

wish to navigate this hierarchy, you could search Yahoo to see if the term 'Midwifery' existed in the subject catalogue. Either way, you end up at the same point (Fig. 3.7).

- From the 'Midwifery' subject category, six Internet resources are suggested. These range from very specific resources, such as a link to a site concerned with the safety of home births, to more general sites such as the 'Online Birth Centre' where numerous resources of interest to practising midwives can be found (Fig. 3.8).
If your Web browser has been set up to read Usenet News articles, Yahoo also includes a link to the *sci.med.midwifery* newsgroup. Following this link will enable you to browse through the recent discussions that have taken place in this midwifery focused newsgroup. Chapter 6 gives further details of Usenet News.

Comment
Though the resources identified in this search do not represent the total of all midwifery resources, they nevertheless provide the midwife with an excellent starting point.

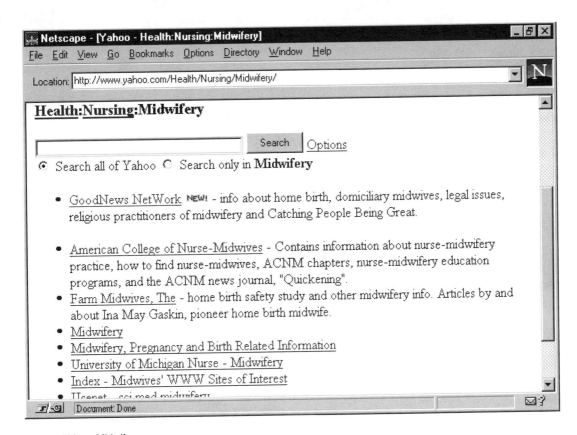

Fig. 3.7   Yahoo: Midwifery

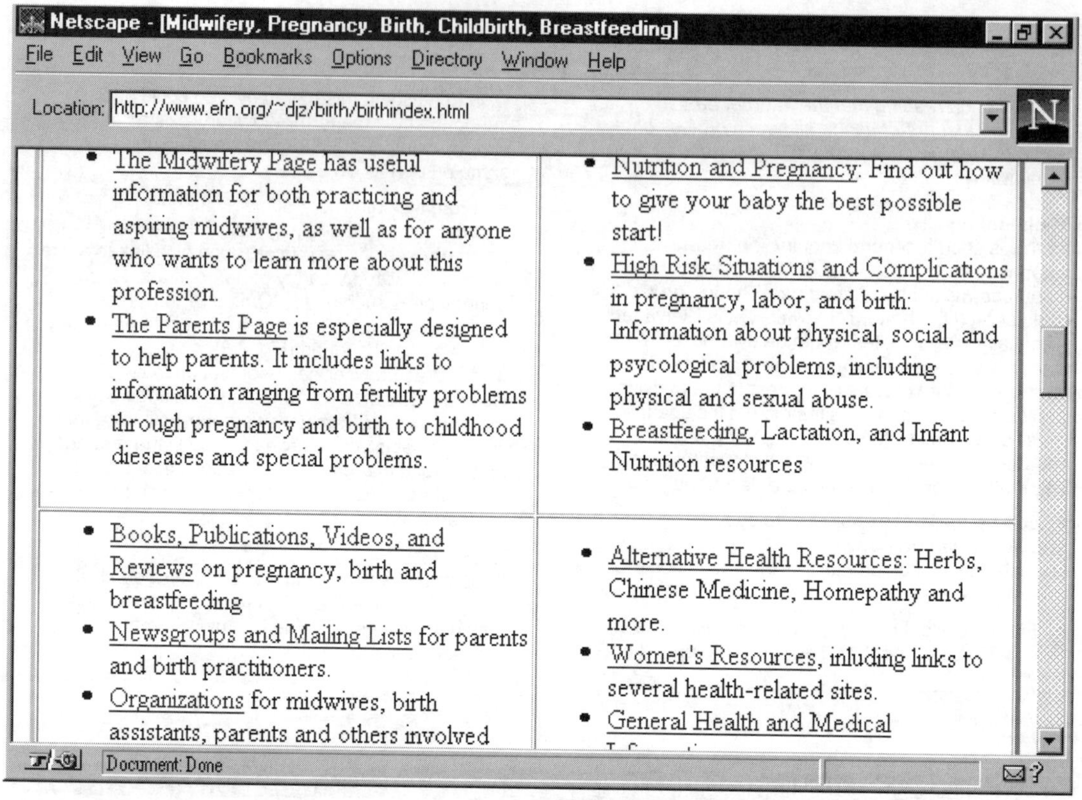

Netscape - [Midwifery, Pregnancy, Birth, Childbirth, Breastfeeding]

File Edit View Go Bookmarks Options Directory Window Help

Location: http://www.efn.org/~djz/birth/birthindex.html

- The Midwifery Page has useful information for both practicing and aspiring midwives, as well as for anyone who wants to learn more about this profession.
- The Parents Page is especially designed to help parents. It includes links to information ranging from fertility problems through pregnancy and birth to childhood dieseases and special problems.

- Books, Publications, Videos, and Reviews on pregnancy, birth and breastfeeding
- Newsgroups and Mailing Lists for parents and birth practitioners.
- Organizations for midwives, birth assistants, parents and others involved

- Nutrition and Pregnancy: Find out how to give your baby the best possible start!
- High Risk Situations and Complications in pregnancy, labor, and birth: Information about physical, social, and psycological problems, including physical and sexual abuse.
- Breastfeeding, Lactation, and Infant Nutrition resources

- Alternative Health Resources: Herbs, Chinese Medicine, Homepathy and more.
- Women's Resources, inluding links to several health-related sites.
- General Health and Medical

Document: Done

Fig. 3.8 Midwifery resources

EVALUATED SUBJECT CATALOGUES

The third approach you can use to find medical information is to browse, or search, the growing number of *evaluated* subject catalogues. These have been compiled by individuals, cognisant with the needs of health professionals who only want to find relevant and authoritative sources of information.

Medical Matrix

http://www.slackinc.com/matrix/

Devised by the Internet Working Group of the American Medical Informatics Association, the Medical Matrix is one of the most comprehensive lists of evaluated sources of medical information currently available.

Like Yahoo, each entry in the catalogue has been assigned a subject heading that fits within a hierarchical structure. The 24 top-level subject headings include 'Disease Categorized Information', 'Speciality Categorized Information', 'Clinical Practice Issues', and 'Medical Education'.

For example, on selecting the 'Disease Categorized Information' heading, you are presented with a list of around 20 diseases, including 'AIDS', 'Diabetes' and 'Multiple sclerosis'. Selecting any subject will, in turn, generate a list of Internet resources related to that disease. To focus your search further, the Matrix then arranges the information into subcategories such as Web resources, images, multimedia modules and discussion forums.

In addition to providing the hypertext link to reach the identified resources, the Matrix also gives a description that details what type of information is held at each site. For example, arranged under the 'AIDS' subject heading there is a site entitled 'AIDS Alert for Health Care Workers'.[13] From the Matrix one learns that this is 'an index to journal articles that addresses the occupational health and safety of AIDS health care workers'.

Descriptions such as these benefit the Internet user in two ways. First, they help ensure that your time is not wasted visiting irrelevant sites. Secondly, because less time is spent 'surfing' the Internet – often in a desperate attempt to find an appropriate resource – the total traffic on the Network is reduced. Like any highway, the less traffic using it the quicker you reach your destination. In terms of the Internet, this means that data are delivered to your desktop more quickly, and less time is spent reading the 'waiting for host to respond' status message.

The Matrix is also an excellent site for keeping up-to-date with new health-related Internet resources. Simply follow the links under the 'What's New?' heading, or join the discussion list *mmatrix-l* by sending the e-mail shown in Figure 3.9. Chapter 6 gives full details on how to send e-mails.

To:	listserv@kumchttp.mc.ukans.edu
Subject:	*leave blank*
Text:	subscribe mmatrix-l *firstname surname*

Fig. 3.9   Joining the *mmatrix-l* discussion list

OMNI

http://www.omni.ac.uk

OMNI stands for Organised Medical Network Information. In many ways, the OMNI project can be seen as the UK equivalent to the Medical Matrix. Like the Matrix, each resource added to the OMNI database includes a short description that allows you decide in advance whether or not it will provide the information you require. Secondly, only resources that have been quality assessed are included. Thirdly, each entry to the database is assigned a subject heading.

OMNI differs, however, in that the database can also be searched by keyword. This is done through an uncluttered World Wide Web search-query form (Fig. 3.10).

It is worth noting that the indexing thesaurus used by OMNI is the National Library of Medicine's Medical Subject Headings (MeSH). Thus, to identify 'cancer' resources you must use the preferred MeSH term 'oncology'. If you are unfamiliar with this thesaurus, you may find the browsing option more appropriate.

At the time of writing, OMNI is still very much in its developmental stage. However, its explicit commitment to providing a gateway to *quality* resources, coupled with its acknowledged bias to UK Internet sites (a counterbalance to the US bias of the Medical Matrix), should ensure that OMNI becomes an indispensable tool for all health professionals.

CliniWeb

http://www.ohsu.edu/cliniweb/

This resource, developed by the Oregon Health Sciences University, also allows physicians and clinicians to search for information by subject. CliniWeb differs from both the Medical Matrix and OMNI in that it indexes information at the level of *individual pages* on the World Wide Web. For example, whereas OMNI provides a link to the CHORUS Database Home Page, staff at CliniWeb have indexed individual documents within this database.[14] Thus, a search on CliniWeb for the term 'tuberculosis' points you to a specific document on the CHORUS database about the gastrointestinal manifestations of this disease. The same search on OMNI does not identify this resource, or even suggest CHORUS as a possible site for this subject.

As with any type of literature searching, the key factor in determining whether or not the search will be successful – that is, retrieve highly relevant documents – is whether or not the correct subject headings are used. To assist in this task, CliniWeb have employed a program called SAPHIRE that maps free-text, natural language terms, to the correct MeSH term. For example, the user can input a phrase such as 'coronary heart bypass surgery', and

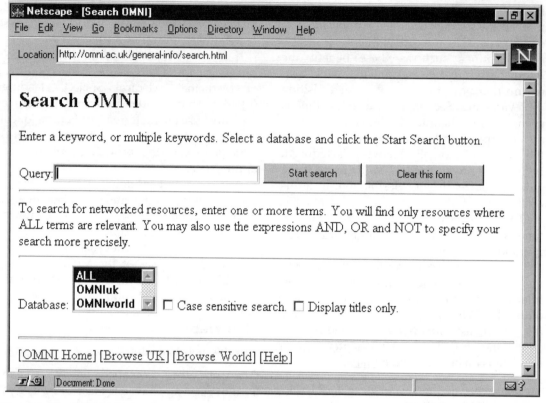

Fig. 3.10 The OMNI search interface

allow SAPHIRE to map it to the correct subject heading, 'Coronary Disease'. In this example, a selection of Web sites were identified, including a link to an article in the *British Medical Journal* entitled, 'Volume and outcome in coronary artery bypass graft surgery'.[15] Clicking on this link takes you to the *BMJ* site, where you can read an abstract of this article, along with the full bibliographic citation.

Appropriate subject headings can also be identified by browsing the MeSH hierarchical structure. Via this method, subject headings are expanded and contracted until the desired term is identified. Figure 3.11 demonstrates the hierarchical nature of MeSH on CliniWeb.

Though it would be going too far to say that every URL identified by CliniWeb has been peer-reviewed, and is therefore an authoritative source, the developers of CliniWeb have at least begun to address this issue. Their claim that 'pages not dealing with clinical topics at the level of students or providers were

deliberately not indexed' is tacit recognition of the importance of critically assessing Web pages.[16]

At the present moment CliniWeb is relatively small. The 2500 URLs in the database

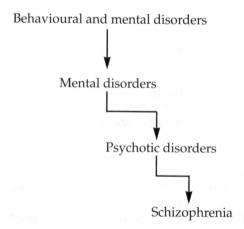

Fig. 3.11 MeSH hierarchy on CliniWeb: progression from broad to narrow concepts

seems insignificant when compared to something like MEDLINE, which in the last 5 years alone has indexed more than 1.6 million documents. However, the fact that the CliniWeb developers have decided to index the clinical resources of the Internet at a very detailed level, leads me to believe that, in the future, this will also become an invaluable resource for health professionals.

CIC HealthWeb

http://www.ghsl.nwu.edu/healthweb

The last evaluated subject catalogue to be considered is HealthWeb. Developed by a team of US health science librarians, the aim of this project is to 'develop an interface that will provide organised access to health related Internet accessible resources'.[17]

In practice, a named university takes responsibility for identifying, and assessing Internet resources on a selected subject. Thus the University of Michigan has taken responsibility for identifying information relating to nursing, whilst the University of Indiana is concerned with radiology sources. An alphabetical list of all the subjects covered is available from the HealthWeb Home Page.

Each site sub-divides its specific subject into manageable chunks. The 'Nursing' divisions include 'Career Information', 'Clinical Nursing', 'Research' and 'Resources.' Like the Medical Matrix and OMNI, each resource is annotated to ensure that you only follow useful and relevant links.

The only criticism that can be levelled at HealthWeb is that, like the Virtual Library, there is little uniformity in the way the identified resources are arranged. For example, the Nursing Page categorises nursing journals as a 'Resource'. Follow the links under this heading and you will gain access to journals such as the *American Journal of Nursing* and *Midwifery Today*. To find radiology journals from the Radiology Page, however, one has to follow the 'Electronic Publications' link. This inconsistent approach means that the user has to second-guess where a particular type of resource may be located within the HealthWeb hierarchy.

Summary of evaluated subject catalogues

- For a good overview and introduction to evaluated sources of medical information, use the Medical Matrix.

- If you wish to identify quality British resources, use OMNI.

- To identify specific documents, rather than resources of a more general nature, use CliniWeb.

- To identify high-quality resources for the professions allied to medicine (physical therapy, nursing, etc.) and for the interdisciplinary sciences (minority health, alternative medicine, etc.), use HealthWeb.

Strengths of evaluated subject catalogues

- As the resources are evaluated by professionals *before* they are included in the subject catalogue, highly relevant and qualitative sources of information can be identified quickly and easily.

- The short descriptions that accompany most resource entries enable you to decide in advance whether or not a particular site will provide the information you require.

Weaknesses of evaluated subject catalogues

- Because the catalogues are compiled by individuals, potentially useful resources can be overlooked. For example, the Medical Matrix suggests just *one* asthma resource, the Asthma Patient Teaching Guide.[18] In contrast, a Lycos search on asthma finds numerous sites including the authoritative American Academy of Allergy, Asthma and Immunology, [19] the interesting AsmaNet[20] and the useful Asthma and Allergy WWW Resources Page.[21]

- Most evaluated subject catalogues are still very much in their infancy, and consequently the number of resources identified thus far is quite small.

Using an evaluated subject catalogue

In Box 3.4 is a worked example of using an evaluated subject catalogue to help in responding to a patient's query.

Box 3.4 Using an evaluated subject catalogue: a worked example

A patient, about to undergo a heart bypass operation asks his general practitioner for some information that explains, in layman's terms, the nature of this operation. Can the Internet help?

Methodology
Though it would be possible to do a free-text search on 'heart surgery' or 'bypass operations', it is likely that this would generate a massive number of hits. Moreover, the GP would then have to assess each one to see if they were suitable. To overcome these problems, a specialised, peer-reviewed Internet medical subject catalogue can be consulted. The methodology for doing this is set out below.

* Call up the Medical Matrix:
http://www.slackinc.com/matrix/
I selected this site as all the suggested links in it have been assessed and selected by the American Medical Informatics Association.

* Select the option to view the Matrix by 'Speciality Categorized Internet Information'.

* Select the 'Cardiovascular Surgery' link.

* The Cardiovascular Surgery Page lists various resources including the promising 'Heart Surgery Forum' (Fig. 3.12). The description offered by Medical Matrix is that this site is an 'information hub for practising heart surgeons'.

* Select this link:
http://www.hsforum.com/heartsurgery/homehsf.html
* As you scroll through the table of contents you observe a section entitled 'For non-surgeons' with a link to 'Coronary Artery Bypass Grafting' – a featured educational forum about coronary artery surgery for the lay public – plus a link to a more general discussion on heart disease.

* Select the first of these options:
http://www.hsforum.com/heartsurgery/TLC/CABG/CABGTLC.html
From this link you are given an introduction to the disease and the surgical procedures (Figs 3.13, 3.14). You are also able to look at coronary angiograms, and read about and see a heart-lung machine. Finally, you are given details of outcomes and guidelines on when you can pursue your normal daily activities.

Comment
This example demonstrates that using a specialised Internet subject index can be an excellent way of finding relevant, authoritative documents in a very short space of time. From the first link to the Medical Matrix to the delivery of the document on the desktop, just four mouse-clicks were made.

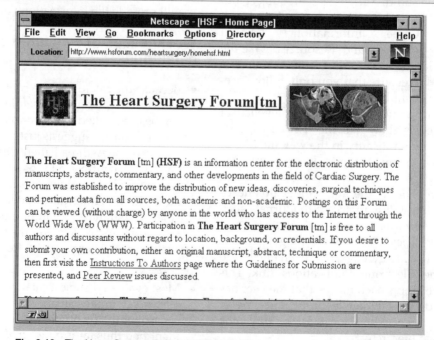

Fig. 3.12 The Heart Surgery Forum (HSF) Home Page

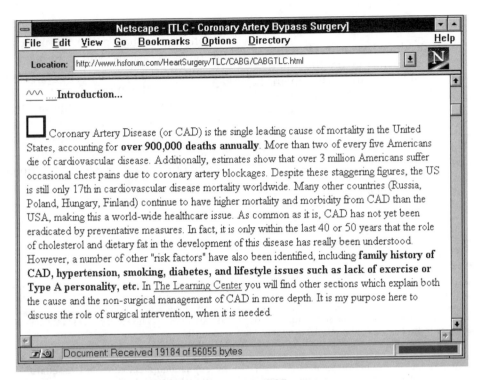

Fig. 3.13 Details of coronary artery disease from the HSF

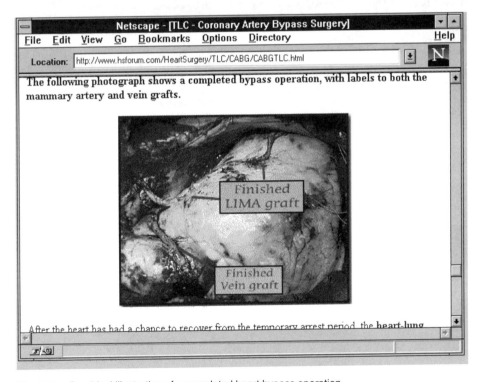

Fig. 3.14 Graphical illustration of a completed heart bypass operation

CONCLUSION

This chapter introduced you to the range of search tools now available on the Internet. Which tool(s) you use will, in the main, be determined by the nature of the search question and by what you hope to find. When you seek just a few high-quality resources, the evaluated subject catalogues will be your best starting point. To get a broader perspective of the information that is available, a general subject catalogue may be of most use. When highly specific resources are sought, a free-text search engine may prove the most effective. On other occasions, you may need to use a combination of these tools before you successfully retrieve the information you require.

As the resources on the Internet are so vast, you can be fairly sure that no matter how obscure your subject interest is, someone, somewhere, will have posted some information about it. With the tools described in this chapter you can find that information.

REFERENCES AND NOTES

1 A Web robot is a computer program that automatically and systematically accesses Web servers to identify what information is available. When this information has been gleaned, the robot 'moves' to the next server. In this sense, the robot 'wanders'. In reality, the program never leaves the host computer.

2 All HTML files comply to a uniform standard, which includes defining a 'header field'. To see the contents of this field in any World Wide Web document, select **Edit | View | Source | Option**. The text between the switches <HEAD> and </head> is defined as the header text.

3 http://www.lycos.cs.cmu.edu/reference.html

4 Other databases of Internet resources that can be searched include:
Alta Vista   http:// www.altavista.com/
Web Crawler   http://www.webcrawler.com/
Inktomi   http://www.inktomi.com/

5 http://neurosurgery.mgh.harvard.edu/paral-r.htm

6 http://www.well.com/user/bengston/pages.pcpc.htm

7 http://www.motorcycle.com/mo/mctext/rzstory.html

8 http://cancer.med./upenn.edu/

9 http://www.nci.nih.gov/

10 Anonymous Hide and go seek. PC Computing 1995 8 (9):167

11 http://golgi.harvard.edu/htbin/biopages

12 http://www.cdc.gov/

13 gopher://gopher.cic.net: 70/11/e-serials/alphabetic/a/aids-alert

14 CHORUS – a searchable collection of documents on diseases and syndromes:
http://chorus.rad.mcw.edu/chorus.html

15 http://www.cityscape.co.uk/users/dl88/archive/6998a.htm#1

16 http://www.ohsu.edu/cliniweb/about.html

17 http://www.ghsl.nwu.edu/healthweb/about.html

18 http://www.meddean.luc.edu/lumen/MedEd/Medicine/Allergy/Asthma/asthtoc.html

19 http://execpc.com/~edi/aaaai.html

20 http://www.remcomp.com/asmanet/asmanet.html

21 http://www.cco.caltech.edu/~wrean/resources.html

4

The top ten medical resources

Box 4.1 Chapter objectives

- Introduce you to some of the premier health and medical resources on the Internet.
- Provide detailed descriptions of these resources.
- Illustrate by case-study how these resources can be used to answer specific medical queries.

INTRODUCTION

One of the best metaphors for the Internet I have come across likened this large and sprawling network to a city. Like any city, the Internet has many useful and interesting places to visit. It also provides opportunities to buy and sell products and, in common with other cities, has a seedier and darker side that is best left uncharted.

To find your way around, street maps and signposts are required, which in Internet terms equate to <u>search engines</u> and <u>subject catalogues</u> (Ch. 3). New visitors, however, may wish to supplement their 'A to Z' with a tourist guide that readily identifies some of the best places to visit. With this analogy in mind, this chapter can be seen as your starting point for Internet exploration.

In keeping with the tradition set by all good travel guides, every place (site) identified has a map reference – a <u>URL</u> – and a detailed description of the available resources. To keep the discussion focused on how the Internet can help in your day-to-day clinical work, the descriptions of every site also include a case study demonstrating how a specific medical query was answered by that resource.

By providing this information in an off-line format, this chapter will help you identify useful resources before logging-on, and will help develop your appreciation of the wealth of information that awaits you.

As the Internet is such a dynamic and ever-changing entity, there is always the danger that any resource list will be out-of-date before it has been published. To negate this threat, emphasis has been placed on the type of information a particular server holds rather than on specific elements of data. For example, it is possible that the World Health Organization (WHO) may delete the information it currently holds on the incidence of malaria. What the WHO is far less likely to do is to remove *all* the resources relating to statistical information. Thus, if you are seeking global and authoritative statistical data, the WHO will always be a good starting point.

ACCESS

The top ten medical resources identified in this chapter can be accessed from the Churchill Livingstone World Wide Web page. This single access point not only simplifies your Internet exploration – by making the typing of long and complicated URLs unnecessary – but more importantly, if any of the URLs cited in this chapter change in any way, the new addresses will be recorded and made available to you from this Web page.

To reach Churchill Livingstone's Medical Information on the Internet page, point your Web browser at the following location:

http://www.churchillmed.com/BOOKS/ medinter.html

It is recommended that you bookmark this page or even make it your default Home Page (Appendix B).

Selection criteria

It would be nice to say that all of the sites described below were selected by the application of some strict, internationally recognised, quality criteria. Unfortunately, there is no BS5750-type standard that one can employ.

Indeed, the only time quality marks are awarded is when organisations such as Point Communications ask users to vote for the 'best Web sites'. In these surveys though, marks are awarded more for presentation and for 'new uses of the Web' than for the content of the available material.

Consequently, in drawing up my list of 'places to visit' I have devised my own selection criteria. Thus I have:

- given pointers to information providers whose contributions to the knowledge base of medicine has long been recognised as authoritative. The Centers for Disease Control and Prevention (CDC), and the World Health Organization are just two examples of "publishers" who have made a considerable impact on the the Internet;

- included a mix of resources that can be used to answer a variety of information queries;

- included a range of different *types* of information. Some sites are purely textual, others may have a mix of text and graphics, or be in the form of a database which you can search;

- excluded sites that are not regularly updated. The Primary Health Care Guide[1] for example, started off as a most promising Web site. It has been excluded from the list as its Web pages have become very dated;

- excluded sites whose primary focus is medical education – this is looked at in Chapter 5;

- excluded sites that are just pointers to other resources. Thus in this list there is no place for sites such as OMNI or HealthWeb. (Ch. 3);

- excluded sites that cannot be reached through a standard Web browser, or Helper Applications like Telnet. Thus, the *Cochrane Database of Systematic Reviews* is excluded as access is restricted to users of the JANUS Internet Medical Browser.

THE 'MEDICAL TOP TEN'

In restricting this list to just ten Internet sites, I have inevitably omitted many valuable resources. Those that *have* made it into this list are, in my opinion, the most useful Internet sites currently available for health professionals, and ones that will be accessed time and time again. They are listed in Box 4.2 in alphabetical order as further ranking would be invidious.

Only one of the top ten sites is based in the UK – the NHS Centre for Reviews and Dissemination. This situation reflects the cautious – or ambivalent – attitude the medical authorities in this country have adopted towards the Internet. To date, not a single UK Royal College has ventured on to the Internet. The same is true for the influential health bodies such as the Kings Fund or the Nuffield Institute for Health.

Similarly, key publications such as the *British National Formulary* (*BNF*) or the *Medical Register* have yet to appear in this medium. Though in recent months the Department of Health has started to develop a range of Web pages,[2] the paucity of hard information at this site leads some cynics to conclude that it is more a public relations exercise than a serious attempt to inform.

In drawing attention to this situation, and contrasting it with the wealth of medical information other countries (notably the USA) make available, I hope to encourage the UK medical community to take up the opportunity that the Internet offers. Whether it is disseminating research findings or demonstrating examples of good practice, the Internet is the *only* medium where a truly world-wide audience can be assured.

The case studies below should also dispel any notion that the Internet is just a 'plaything' or 'this year's gimmick', and demonstrate instead its relevance and importance to the medical community.

Box 4.2   The 'medical top ten'

- Cable News Network Food and Health Page
- Centers for Disease Control and Prevention
- The National Institutes of Health
- The National Library of Medicine
- NHS Centre for Reviews and Dissemination
- OncoLink
- Physicians GenRx
- Physicians Home Page
- UnCover
- The World Health Organization

Cable News Network Food and Health News Page

http://www.cnn.com/HEALTH/index.html

Resources Discussion and analysis of today's health issues as reported by Cable News Network (CNN).

Cost Free.

Analysis Though the CNN site may seem an unlikely candidate for this list of top ten medical sites, it is an excellent resource for health professionals who wish to be kept aware of health stories – and scares – as they break in the press and on television.

Updated daily, this site usually contains one or two main stories, plus half-a-dozen 'health briefs'. On the day I wrote this piece, the lead story looked at cholesterol screening in the light of a recently published report.

What clearly differentiates the CNN health pages from a range of other 'news-wire' services is the fact that each lead story is sprinkled with hypertext links to related sites. Thus, in the cholesterol example, there was a link to the American Heart Association,[3] the *Nutrition Expert Home Page*,[4] and by way of providing a balance to this coverage, there was also a link to an article held on a server at Dundee University entitled, 'Cholesterol screening: can it be justified?'[5]

Each story is further enhanced by CNN's extensive use of graphics, moving images and sound clips. If you have not yet experienced the true multimedia nature of the Internet, the CNN pages are a revelation

For an illustration of how this resource was used to answer a medical query see Box 4.3.

Box 4.3 Case study for CNN

A patient contacts his general practitioner requesting further details of a story, heard on the radio that morning, that a new drug has been identified that may help AIDS patients.

Methodology
For topical information such as this, the CNN site will always be a good starting point. On accessing the *CNN Health Home Page*, a quick scan of the 'top stories' reveals the headline '*Drug may boost immunity for AIDS* patient' (Fig. 4.1).[6] By linking to this story, the GP discovers that the new drug is ritonavir (ABT 538) and that it

will made available, by lottery, for 2000 people. This page also indicates that the original research that sparked this story was published in this week's *New England Journal of Medicine* (*NEJM*). When this journal becomes available over the Internet, it can be assumed that CNN will provide a direct link to the specific article at the *NEJM* site.

The CNN article concludes with links to other AIDS reports from the CNN library, plus links to the National AIDS Clearinghouse,[7] the CDC,[8] and the *AIDS Information Newsletter*.[9]

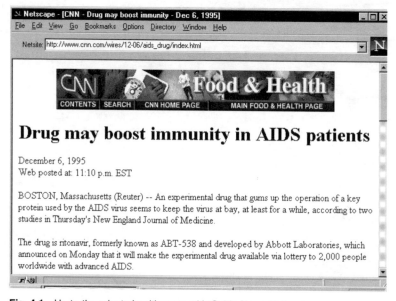

Fig. 4.1 Up-to-the minute health news with Cable News Network

Centers for Disease Control and Prevention

http://www.cdc.gov/

Resources The Centers for Disease Control and Prevention (CDC) is *the* site to visit if you are looking for information on chronic diseases, injuries and disabilities, or guidelines on their prevention.

In addition to these sources, the CDC has valuable data on travellers health, plus full-text access to the *Morbidity and Mortality Weekly Report* (MMWR).

Cost   Free.

Analysis   The stated aim of the CDC is to 'promote health and quality of life by preventing and controlling disease, injury and disability'.[10] In addressing this broad agenda, the CDC has developed numerous information resources of use and interest to all health professionals. Fortunately, many of the resources held at CDC can be accessed through one sophisticated search tool, known as CDC WONDER.

CDC WONDER provides query access to about 40 text and numerical databases. For example, when you select the mortality data-set, to retrieve data on the causes of death, you can define your search parameters to include a particular state, race, gender or age. Text databases such as the *Prevention Guidelines* and *MMWR* can be searched by keyword.

For information about travellers health, CDC provide a hypertext map of the world (Fig. 4.2). By pointing and clicking your mouse on a particular country you can identify its current vaccine requirements, details of any prevalent diseases, plus general health and travel advice. This type of information is updated frequently to take account of recently reported disease outbreaks.

For an illustration of how this resource was used to answer a medical query see Box 4.4.

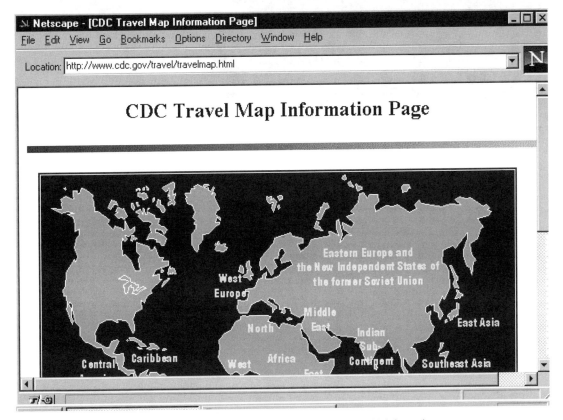

Fig. 4.2   The CDC hypertext map of the world: point and click for travellers' health information

---

Box 4.4 Case study for CDC

A hospital microbiologist, concerned by the large number of TB cases he has seen in recent months, contacts the library to see if there are any current documents examining the prevention and control of this disease.

Methodology
As the CDC is probably the world's leading authority on disease prevention, contacting its Internet site is a logical decision.

At the CDC Home Page there is a link entitled 'Prevention Guidelines' that takes the microbiologist to Prevention Guidelines, a database described as

a 'comprehensive compendium of all guidelines and recommendations produced by the CDC'.[11]

Though this database does not support free-text searching, it can be browsed by title or topic. From the 'topic' link, an alphabetical list of keywords is displayed. On selecting 'tuberculosis', around 20 titles, in reverse chronological order, are presented on your screen. As the documents *Essential components of a tuberculosis prevention and control program* (1995),[12] and *Guidelines for preventing the transmission of mycobacterium tuberculosis in health care facilities* (1994)[13] seem particularly pertinent to this enquiry, they can be FTPd (Fig. 4.3).

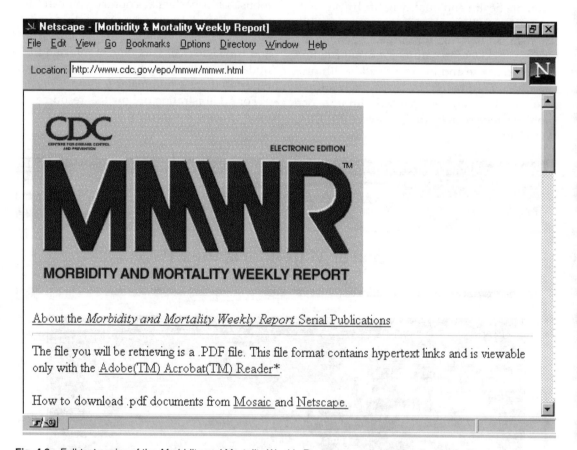

Fig. 4.3 Full-text copies of the *Morbidity and Mortality Weekly Report* are available from the CDC site

National Institutes of Health

http://www.nih.gov

Resources The National Institutes of Health (NIH) supply Consensus Development Statements; information about cancer and its treatment (Cancer-Net); AIDS resources; and details of current research activities.

Cost Free.

Analysis Recognised among the world's foremost biomedical research centres, the National Institutes of Health provide a range of invaluable sources of information for health professionals.

The Consensus Development Conferences, and the subsequent Statements are authoritative guides to current medical issues. Scanning the titles of some of the most recent *Statements* – on physical therapy and cardiovascular disease, ovarian cancer screening, and cochlear implants – demonstrates the commitment of the NIH to focus on mainstream clinical issues.

The Cancer-Net Service, developed by the National Cancer Institute (NCI), provides fact sheets on topics such as cancer detection, prevention and therapy. It is also possible to perform a literature search on the *Cancer-Net* database to identify specific references. A search on 'HRT' for example, found a document on breast cancer that included detailed analysis of the effect of HRT on this disease. Moreover, as it was authored by the NCI, its findings can be assumed to be an accurate reflection of current medical opinion on this subject.

One other very useful resource is the NIH Information Index which it identifies those diseases currently being researched by NIH scientists. Searchable by keyword, it is possible to enter a term such as 'asthma' and find out if any NIH departments are researching this disease. If you are about to undertake a major piece of research, using this resource *first* will ensure that you do not waste time and resources repeating work that is already being undertaken. It also serves as an ideal way to make contact with fellow specialists.

For an illustration of how this resource was used to answer a medical query see Box 4.5.

Box 4.5   Case study for NIH

A consultant orthopaedic surgeon wishes to know which surgical technique for total hip replacement produces the best long-term outcomes.

Methodology
Though a <u>MEDLINE</u> search would normally be the starting point for such an enquiry, the surgeon's knowledge of this database suggests that this type of search will generate hundreds of 'hits'. What is required is one document that will compare the different surgical techniques and, more importantly, indicate which method produces the best outcomes.

As hip replacements are a relatively common procedure, it is a reasonable assumption that the NIH will have discussed it. From the *NIH Health Information Home Page* there is a link to all the *NIH Consensus Statements*. At this point, the surgeon can either employ a search engine, which will search the entire contents of every published *Consensus Statement*, or browse the Statement titles. Either way identifies the Consensus Statement *Total Hip Replacement* (Fig. 4.4). From this page, the surgeon can jump to a detailed 'Table of contents' that includes 'What are the design and surgical considerations relating to replacement prosthesis'.[14] Either this section, or the whole Statement, can be FTP'd.

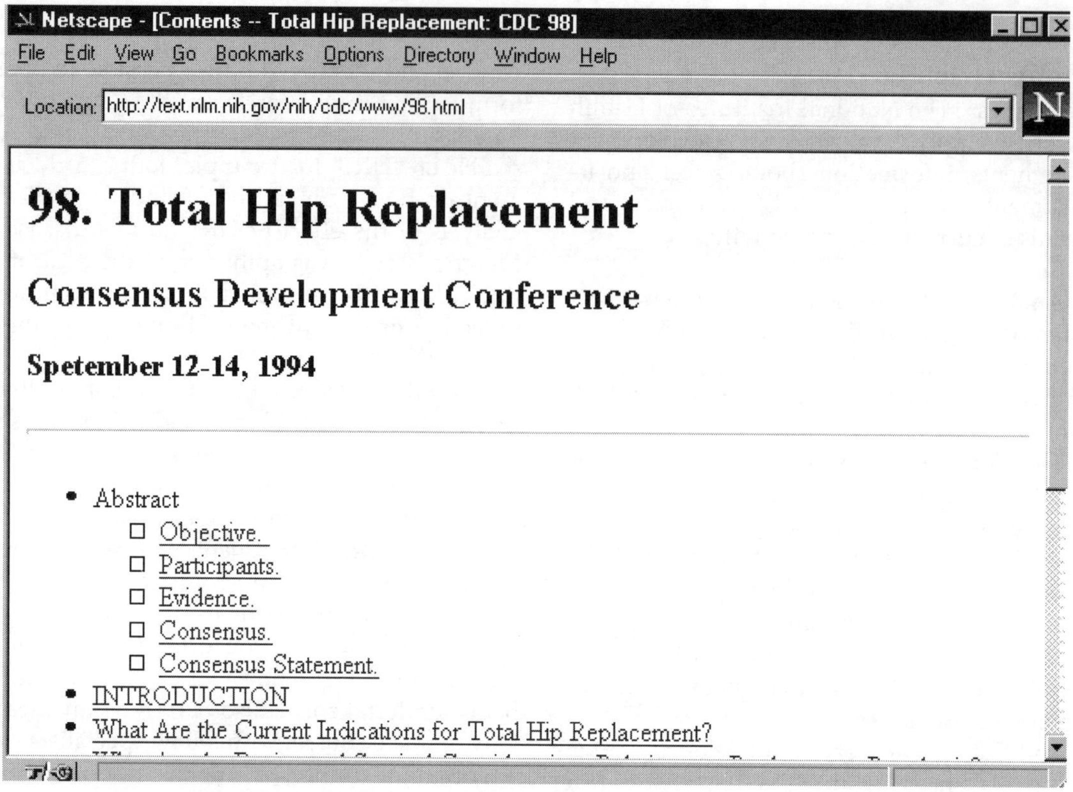

Fig. 4.4 Consensus Statement from the NIH

National Library of Medicine

http://www.nlm.nih.gov/

Note Though part of the National Institutes of Health, the National Library of Medicine (NLM) has its *own* entry in this resource list to reflect the wealth of health information available at this site.

Resources AIDS databases; Visible Human Project; the NLM book and audio-visual catalogue; access to the Agency for Health Policy and Research (AHCPR) clinical practice guidelines; and a large selection of images from the History of Medicine Division.

Cost Free.

Analysis Though the NLM does not yet offer non-US customers direct access to MED-LINE (the most popular biomedical database in the world is produced by this organisation), this site still has a wide range of useful resources for health professionals. MEDLINE access is discussed under '*Physicians Home Page*' (below).

Researchers involved in the detection, prevention and treatment of AIDS will find the AIDSLINE, AIDSDRUGS and AIDSTRIALS databases essential reference points. Following a resolution passed at a recent NIH conference, these databases are available without charge.

Of more general use is the NLM *Locator Catalog*. Containing around 5 million items this database can be searched to see what books or audio-visuals are held by the library. Though borrowing from this source is prohibited, once you know *what* exists on your speciality, you can see if your hospital library has it or can obtain it from a more local source.

The NLM has also developed a full-text database (HSTAT) that gives access to the AHCPR clinical guidelines, NIH consensus statements and other key protocol-based documents. The NLM is also the body responsible for distributing NIH findings 'which could immediately benefit human morbidity and mortality'.[15] To access these 'Alerts' go to:

gopher://gopher.nlm.nih.gov: 70/11/alerts

The *Visible Human Project* is a long-term plan by the NLM to build a digital image library consisting of complete, anatomically detailed, three-dimensional representations of the male and female human (Fig. 4.5). The current phase of the project is collecting trans-verse CAT, MRI and cryosection images of representative male and female cadavers at one millimetre intervals.

Finally, the OnLine Images Database of the History of Medicine Division provide an opportunity to see some unique medical prints and photographs acquired by this department.

For an illustration of how this resource was used to answer a medical query see Box 4.6.

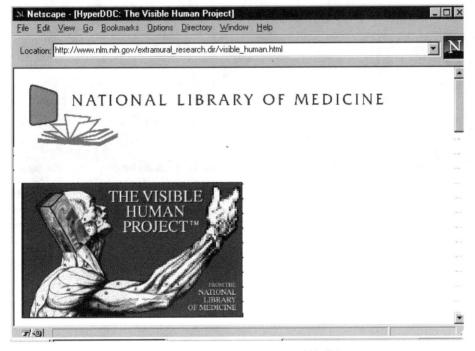

Fig. 4.5 The Visible Human Project from the National Library of Medicine

---

Box 4.6 Case study for NLM

A consultant, devising a presentation on the subject of anaesthesia, decides that a few historical images, showing its use through the ages, will enrich and enliven the talk. Question: Where can you find such pictures?

Methodology
With more than 60 000 prints, the NLM History of Medicine Division probably has the most extensive collection of medical images anywhere in the world. Using its sophisticated search engine, the OnLine Images Database can be searched using free-text expressions. If too many images are retrieved, the search can be narrowed by specifying where the

image originated, and at what date.

In the question posed above, the term 'anesthesia' (US spelling) was combined with a request to limit the search to material that originated in Europe between 1600 and 1900. Thirteen images were retrieved including an 1830 print of a man forcing a bag of laughing gas on a woman – '*Prescription for Scolding Wives*' (Fig. 4.6)[16] – and a picture of a pickpocket using ether to render his victims unconscious.[17]

The selected images can be saved as jpg files and either printed or inserted as a file into the consultant's presentation software. (Microsoft *PowerPoint* and Lotus *Freelance* presentation software are both able to import, and display jpg files.)

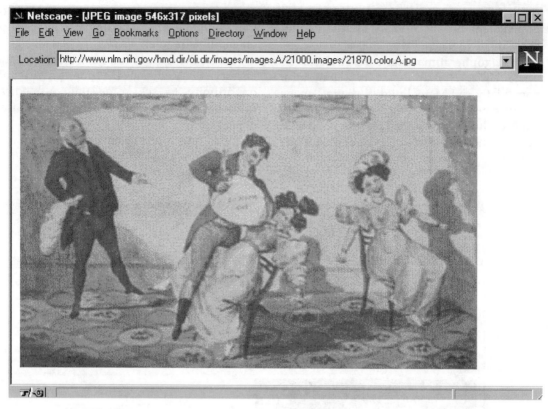

Fig. 4.6 'Prescription for Scolding Wives' © NLM History of Medicine Division

NHS Centre for Reviews and Dissemination (NHS CRD)

http://www.york.ac.uk/inst/crd/info
telnet://nhscrd.york.ac.uk
(ID = crduser; password = crduser)

Resources The NHS Centre for Reviews and Dissemination (NHS CRD) is a database of reviews concerned with the effectiveness and cost-effectiveness of healthcare interventions.

Cost Free.

Analysis Commissioned by the UK NHS Research and Development Division, the purpose of the NHS CRD is to 'identify and review the results of good quality health research and to actively disseminate the findings to key decision makers in the NHS'.[18] As it is estimated that at least £1 billion of National Health Services resources could be released for improving patient care by cutting out unnecessary and ineffective treatments,

awareness of the NHS CRD resource is absolutely essential.[19]

The *Database of Abstracts of Reviews* and *Effectiveness* (DARE) provides structured abstracts of published reviews. These abstracts not only summarise the review but, more importantly, offer a commentary on the rigour with which the research was conducted. Following the recent controversy that symposia published in peer-reviewed medical journals tend to promote the drugs of the sponsoring company unfairly, this unbiased, critical approach is a most welcome and necessary development.[20]

To meet the demand that health care interventions should also be looked at from an economic viewpoint, the CRD has produced the NHS Economic Evaluation Database (NEED). Each record in this database includes a structured summary and an assessment of the *quality* of the economic analysis. This function is undertaken by independent health economists who consider factors such as whether or not the costing methodology is valid and whether or not uncertainties and variables have been properly considered.

Almost all of the citations in the CRD databases can be found on MEDLINE. However, if you are seeking systematic, rigorous and unbiased assessments of published reviews, then the CRD databases should not be overlooked.

For an illustration of how this resource was used to answer a medical query see Box 4.7.

Box 4.7   Case study for NHS CRD

An NHS Trust manager, concerned by the rising cost of the ante-natal service wants to know whether or not the 'triple test' screening for Down's syndrome is cost effective.

Methodology
A search of the NEED database identifies two reviews on this subject. One of these, in the *BMJ*, concludes that the cost of this programme is £28 500 per avoided birth. This contrasts with the accepted cost of caring for a Down's syndrome child of £120 000. With such data, the author concludes that the screening programme is highly cost-effective.[21]

The CRD reviewer, however, is not quite so convinced and identifies a number of weaknesses in the *BMJ* report (Fig. 4.7). The most notable of these is the fact that the original study did not take into account the number of Down's syndrome pregnancies that would have been detected *without* the triple test. In rectifying this, and other omissions, the CDR reviewer calculates that the projected cost of avoided birth should be increased by around 38%.[22]

Though, in this example, the programme is still cost-effective, there will undoubtedly be cases where such an increase in cost brings into question the cost-effectiveness of the intervention.

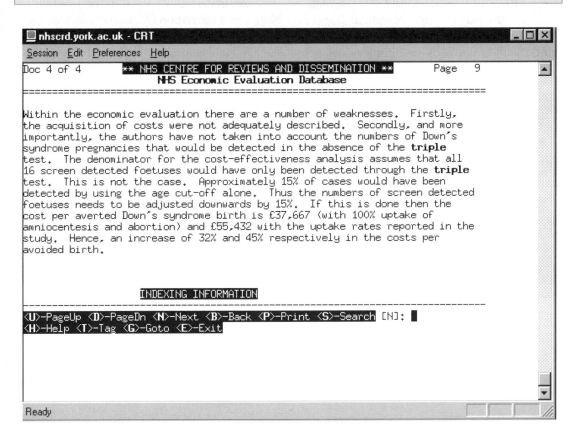

Fig. 4.7   The NHS Centre for Reviews and Dissemination

OncoLink

http://cancer.med.upenn.edu/

Resources Detailed and authoritative information on all aspects of cancer.

Cost Free.

Analysis This site is the only one in this list that is disease-specific. Its inclusion reflects the quality of the information and the ease with which cancer-related questions can be answered.

A clear and simple front menu allows you to approach the resources at OncoLink by eight main categories, including disease, medical speciality (chemotherapy, surgical oncology etc.) and the causes of cancer.

For cancer patients and their families, the Psychological Support Menu provides links to documents that discuss how one can cope with cancer, as well as specific issues such as 'Cancer and sexuality'. In contrast, physicians undertaking research on cancer can link to the Clinical Trials section. Here, all trials currently being conducted by the National Cancer Institute are cited and discussed.

If the subject you are searching for does not lend itself to this menu approach, the OncoLink search engine can be used. This engine supports Boolean logic (malignant *and* melanoma *and* sun) and once a search has been executed, the results are ranked so that the most useful and recent documents appear at the top of the list.

Perhaps the most remarkable aspect of the OncoLink service is that despite the mass of information held at this site, it is very easy to find what you are looking for. Cryptic icons are absent, as are the labyrinthine hierarchies that characterise so many Web sites. Developers of new Web sites would be wise to view OncoLink as an excellent example of how information can be effectively disseminated on the Internet.

In 1994, OncoLink was described as the 'best professional service on the Web';[23] an accolade that was matched in 1995 when it was nominated as a finalist in the prestigious National Information Infrastructure Awards.[24]

For an illustration of how this resource was used to answer a medical query see Box 4.8.

Box 4.8 Case study for OncoLink

A health visitor, preparing for a 'well man clinic' needs some current information on testicular cancer.

Methodology
Though MEDLINE and other biomedical and nursing databases would be able to assist with this query, a visit to OncoLink may find all the information the health visitor requires.

As this example is focusing on a specific type of cancer, the health visitor can use the 'Disease Oriented Menu' option. From this page, cancers are divided by age (child and adult), and then by type. Under the adult list, 16 cancers are cited, including 'genitourinary (male) cancer.' On following this link,

a further sub-menu appears offering information on penile, prostate and testicular cancer. The testicular option allows the health visitor to read (or FTP) the documents *Testicular Self-Examination*,[25] and *HSTAT Screening for Testicular Cancer Guidelines*,[26] as well as listen to an audio clip about this disease (Fig. 4.8).[27]

To identify additional information, the links to the National Cancer Institute/ Physicians Data Query (NCI/PDQ) database can be followed. Documents in this file are available in a full-text form (not just the bibliographic data) and are tagged to indicate at whom the information is aimed.

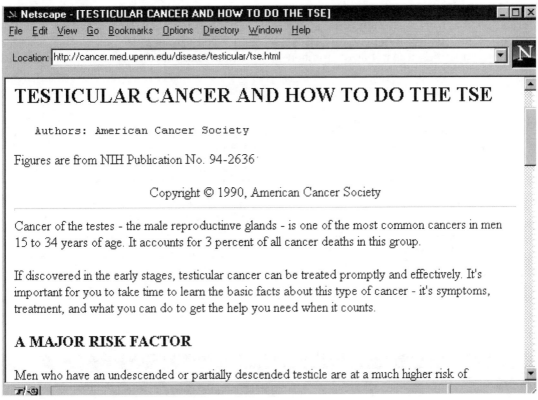

Fig. 4.8   Advice on testicular self-examination from OncoLink

Physicians GenRx

http://www.icsi.net/GenRx

Resources   A database of all prescription pharmaceuticals approved by the Food and Drugs Administration. (FDA).

Costs   A 6-month subscription costs US$89.00; a 12-month subscription US$169.00 (1996 prices). Once your account has been established, there is no restriction on its use.

Analysis   GenRx can be searched in one of two ways. First, by name (either trade or drug) and secondly by category. Via this second option, you can enter a term such as 'antibiotics' or 'antidepressants' and find *all* the drugs in the database which are thus categorised.

As drugs are added to the database, the GenRx team divide each record into 12 unique parts that focus on factors such as 'descrip-

tion', 'warnings', 'precautions' and 'dosage and administration'. This precise structure allows you to configure the results of a search so that you only see the data in which you are interested.

From a UK perspective this database has two minor drawbacks. First, if a drug has a different trade name in the UK from that in the US, then searching by the UK name will retrieve nothing. Secondly, drug prices are quoted in US dollars. However, until the *British National Formulary* (*BNF*) distributes its database over the Internet, then the GenRx product will reign supreme.

For an illustration of how this resource was used to answer a medical query see Box 4.9.

Free alternative and comment   A free

alternative to GenRx is the Pharmaceutical Information Network. Though this source provides high quality independent assessments of therapeutics, it is not as comprehensive, nor as easy to use as GenRx.

This resource can be reached by pointing your Web browser at:

http://pharminfo.com/

Box 4.9   Case study for Physicians GenRx

A general practitioner about to prescribe propranolol to a migraine sufferer wishes to check the literature to ensure that this drug will not interact in any adverse way with the other medication the patient is taking.

Methodology
In a case such as this, the currency and accuracy of the information are the overriding concerns. As the GenRx database is updated regularly, and recognised as a source of unbiased information, using this product makes good clinical sense.[28]

The search on 'propranolol' (Fig. 4.9) is automatically mapped by the database software to the preferred term 'propranolol hydrochloride' (Fig. 4.10). At this point the GP can read (or save to disk) the whole record, or alternatively use the radio-type buttons to focus the search on drug interactions and precautions.

Thus, in a matter of seconds, the GP can be reassured, from the evidence that currently exists, that the prescription he is about to write is clinically valid.

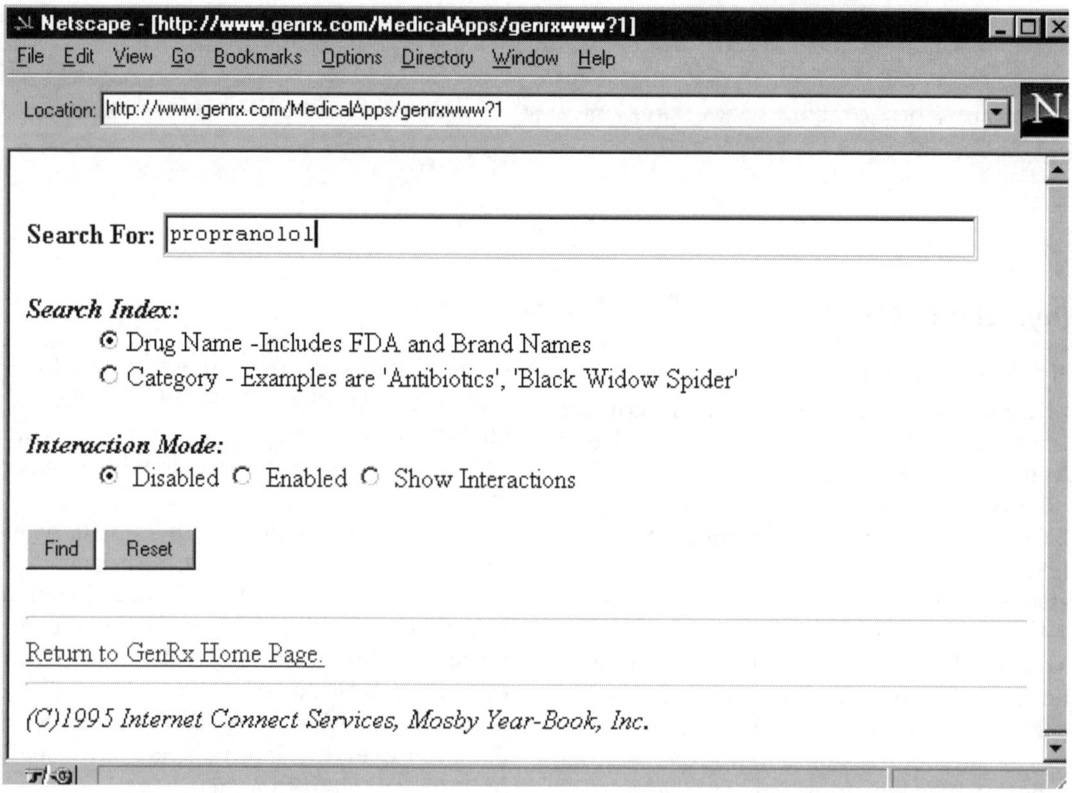

Fig. 4.9 Physicians GenRx search screen

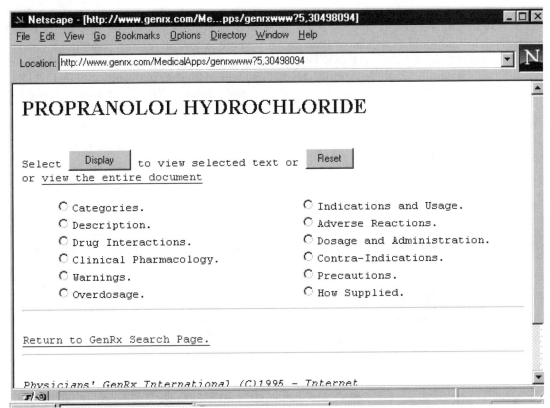

Fig. 4.10 Physicians GenRx results screen: radio-type buttons enable you to customise the results

Physicians Home Page

http://php.silverplatter.com/

Resources This site provides unlimited access to the National Library of Medicine's MEDLINE database, digests of original articles from peer-reviewed medical journals, information about accredited electronic Continuing Medical Education (CME) programmes, plus a conference-like facility where medical questions are posed and discussed.

Costs US$19.95 per month plus an annual international user's fee, as yet unfixed.

Analysis No book about medical information would be complete without some reference to MEDLINE. Incorporating the printed *Index Medicus, International Nursing Index* and the *Index to Dental Literature*, MEDLINE is the largest biomedical bibliographic database. Dating back to 1966, MEDLINE has over

7 million citations, drawn from around 3600 journals. Recent figures indicate that 70% of the citations in the current file include an English abstract.[29]

Searching MEDLINE at the *Physicians Home Page* site is done through a graphical form-based interface – developed by Silver Platter – that you access through your Web browser. On this form you identify your search terms, along with the Boolean operators and any 'limiting' properties you may wish to apply (for example, ensuring that the articles are published in English).

For a more precise search, the MeSH indexing thesaurus can be used. If you are unfamiliar with this, the software can suggest subject headings appropriate to your search. Using this function will, for example, map the term 'heart attack' to the preferred MeSH term 'myocardial infarction'.

The Physicians Home Page is more than just an access point to MEDLINE. The MD Digest service for example, includes 'embedded annotations' that link a user from a summary of one article to other relevant articles in other databases. Where possible, the references cited at the end of the summarised article also have hypertext links to the MEDLINE abstracts.

For an illustration of how this resource was used to answer a medical query see Box 4.10.

Free alternative and comment If your information needs are focused on molecular genetics, then a free subset of MEDLINE – made available by the National Centre for Biotechnology Information (NCBI) – can be found at:

http://www2.ncbi.nlm.nih.gov/medline/ query_form.html

Box 4.10 Case study for Physicians Home Page

A Registrar, preparing for a grand-round presentation, needs to identify some recent articles on the relationship between engine emissions and asthma.

Methodology
At the *Physicians Home Page*, the Registrar selects the option to search MEDLINE. Knowing that searching with MeSH generates fewer irrelevant 'hits' the Registrar asks the software to suggest the most appropriate keywords. 'Asthma' is a MeSH

term and is suggested, whilst 'engine emissions' is mapped to 'automobile-exhaust'. Though, in this example, this term would be selected, it is possible at this point to broaden the search to include all types of air pollution, such as smog and smoke (Fig. 4.11).

The search is further refined to limit the results to those articles which have been published in English within the past 2 years. The resulting list of citations can then be viewed and printed.

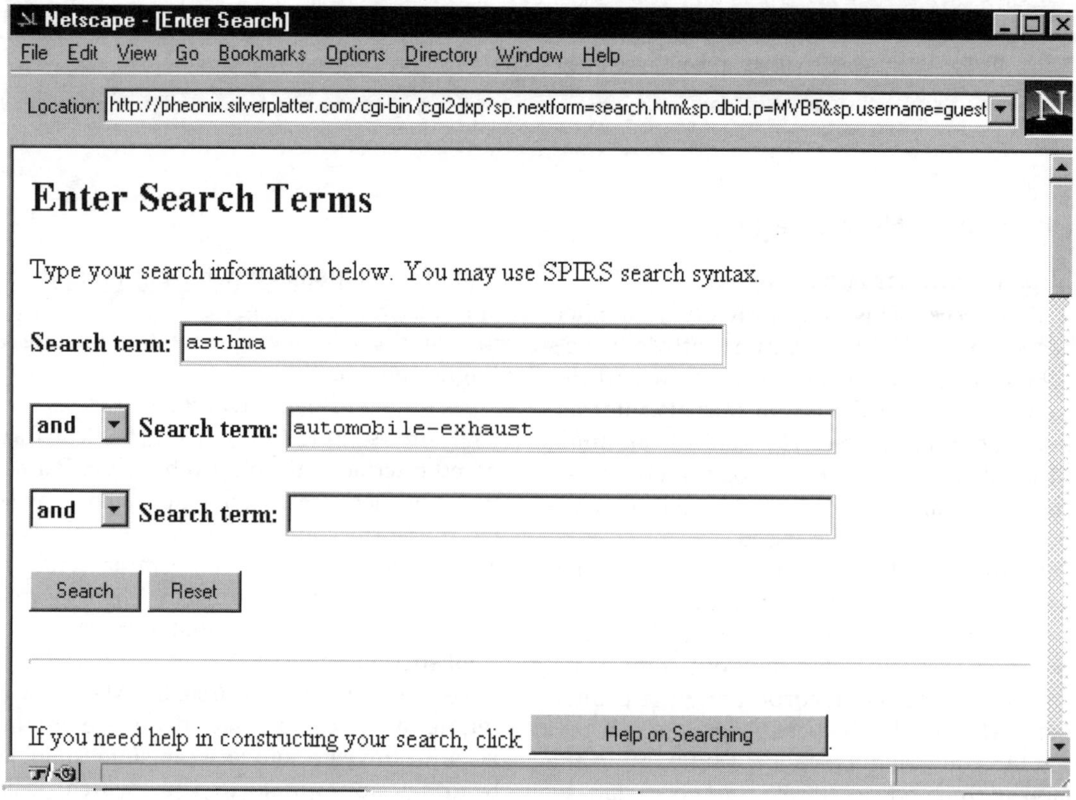

Fig. 4.11 The Physicians Home Page MEDLINE search screen

UnCover

http://www.carl.org/uncover
telnet://database.carl.org

Resources A database of around 6 million journal articles – 4000 citations are added every day – any of which can be faxed to your desktop within 24 hours.

Cost Free to search – other services charged. See below for details.

Analysis Though *UnCover* covers all subject disciplines there has been a concerted effort to address the needs of health professionals. Of the 17 000 journal titles that *UnCover* currently indexes, 14% (around 2200 titles) are health-related.[30]

As the *UnCover* database can be searched by word, phrase or author, it can be used to check bibliographic references, or even perform fairly crude literature searches. (Though the title and author fields are fully indexed, there is no attempt to subject index any of the articles.) Alternatively, as the database can be browsed by journal title, it is possible to see the contents page of any indexed journal without taking out a subscription. No charge is made to access any of these services.

For an annual fee of US$20.00, however, you can arrange to receive, by e-mail, the table of contents for up to 50 journals as they are published. This fee also includes the option to define up to 25 current awareness keyword searches. Once defined, your keywords are run against the *UnCover* database on a weekly basis, and details of any relevant articles are again mailed to you.

To obtain the full-text copy of any article, you are required to pay a fee of US$8.50, plus royalty fees. (An additional fax surcharge is levied on users who are not resident in the United States or Canada.) Before you actually commit your credit card details, the exact cost in US dollars is displayed. At this time, you still have the option to cancel the transaction. Popular journals are appended with the friendly message that 'this article may be available in your library at no cost to you'.

As *UnCover* indexes the table of contents details at about the same time as the journal is published, it is *the* most up-to-date periodical index available anywhere.

For an illustration of how this resource was used to answer a medical query See Box 4.11.

Box 4.11 Case study for UnCover

A Senior House Officer, hoping to get an article accepted for publication, receives a note from a reviewer asking him if he was aware of some recently published work in the journal Obstetrics and Gynaecology on diabetes insipidus? The SHO, conscious of the fact that this title is not held by the local library, and mindful of the need to read this article as quickly as possible contacts UnCover, the document delivery specialists.

Methodology
The easiest way to search the UnCover database is by keyword. Thus, in this example, keying in the terms 'dia-

betes insipidus obstetrics' should be sufficient to identify the appropriate citation. (The search engine does not allow the user to specify in which field – journal name, article title etc. – the terms should appear.)

From this search six citations were identified (Fig. 4.12). A scan through this list identifies the one referred to by the reviewer, plus a couple of other useful-sounding documents. Once these have been selected, and payment details submitted, the articles will be delivered to the SHO's fax machine within 24 hours.

The combined features of UnCover – article delivery, literature searching, and current awareness – make it a truly useful site for all health professionals.

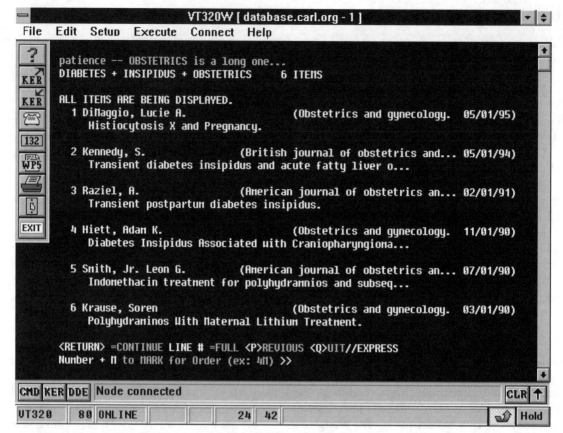

Fig. 4.12 UnCover: results of a search for the terms 'diabetes insipidus obstetrics'

World Health Organization

http://www.who.ch/

Resources Details of World Health Organization (WHO) programmes (Global Programme for Aids, Global Programme for Vaccine and Immunisation etc.); database of WHO publications; statistical databases; *Weekly Epidemiological Report*; press releases and newsletters; access to the *African Index Medicus*.

Cost Free.

Analysis In recognition of the growing importance of the Internet, the WHO have begun to make the *Weekly Epidemiological Report* available via the World Wide Web. This electronic journal provides health professionals with a means of obtaining rapid and accurate epidemiological information and details of new disease outbreaks.

To identify subject-specific WHO resolutions, guidelines, and journal articles, the WHO Library Database (WHOLIS) can be searched. The WHO also provides a statistical service (WHOSIS) giving Internet users access to a variety of data sources such as *Malaria Information Database*, the *Global Health Situation* and *Projects Database*, and the *European Health for all Statistical Database*. The last of these can be FTPd and analysed and manipulated off-line. Work is currently taking place to make the *Mortality Database* available in this fashion.

Recognising the need to improve access to

the health literature published on the African continent, the WHO have also made Internet access possible to the *African Index Medicus*. For researchers looking at health in Africa, this resource should not be overlooked.

If you need a global perspective on health, the WHO Web pages must be seen as *the* essential reference point.

For an illustration of how this resource was used to answer a medical query see Box 4.12.

Box 4.12 Case study for WHO

A general practitioner comments that a large number of people are visiting the surgery with symptoms of influenza. To identify whether or not an outbreak has been officially reported, and if so, whether or not there is any information as to the strain of virus, epidemiological data etc., the WHO server is contacted.

Methodology
Monitoring outbreaks of notifiable diseases has always been one of the primary functions of the WHO. On linking to the WHO server the GP can fol-

low a hypertext link to a page entitled 'Outbreaks' (Fig. 4.13). Selecting this, and bypassing the opportunity to read the latest news concerning the Ebola virus, there is a link to the influenza surveillance activity for the 1995–6 season. This report, compiled by the WHO, is based on reports from National Influenza Centres. The UK entry reports that the influenza is type A(H3N2) and that in November 1995 several health regions reported rates of 178 cases of influenza-like illness per 100 000 population. By the end of January 1996, the figure had fallen to 34.3 per 100 000 population.[31]

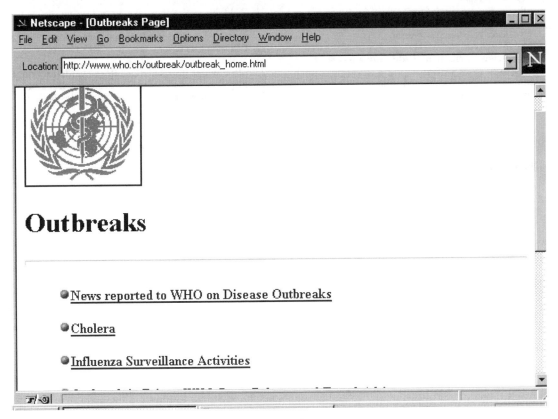

Fig. 4.13 Current disease outbreaks are monitored by the WHO

CONCLUSION

The only way to fully appreciate and exploit the range of resources described in this chapter is to visit these sites and explore. In particular I would urge you to pay particular attention to the *What's New* links. Though at times these may simply serve to distract you from your original objective, on other occasions they will bring to your attention new and useful resources that otherwise would have remained undiscovered.

As you trawl the Internet you will undoubtedly discover numerous other sites of interest and effectively compile your own 'top ten resources'. If you would like to share these findings with other health professionals, please e-mail the details to me through the Churchill Livingstone World Wide Web pages. Subject to the quantity, a 'reader's top ten' will be made available there, along with hypertext links to other recommended sites.

REFERENCES AND NOTES

1 http://www.ukpc.org/
2 http://www.open.gov/doh/dhhome.htm
3 http://www.amhrt.org/
4 http://www.alaska.net:80/~tne
5 http://www.dundee.ac.uk/meded/webupdate/choles/screen.htm
6 http://www.cnn.com/wires/12–06/aids_drug/index.html
7 http://cdcnac.aspensys.com:86/
8 http://www.cdc.gov/
9 http://www.cmpharm.ucsf.edu/~troyer/safesex/vanews
10 http://www.cdc.gov/aboutcdc.htm
11 http://wonder.cdc.gov/wonder/prevguid/prevguid.html
12 http://wonder.cdc.gov/wonder/prevguid/m0038823/m0038823.htm
13 http://wonder.cdc.gov/wonder/prevguid/m0035909/m0035909.htm
14 http://text.nlm.nih.gov/nih/cdc/www/98.html
15 http://cpmcnet.columbia.edu/news/infonews/info0088.html
16 http://www.nlm.nih.gov/cgi-bin/getrec? 571440 Frame 21870 A
17 http://www.nlm.nih.gov/cgi-bin/getrec? 463917 Frame 21634 A
18 http://www.york.ac.uk/inst/crd/welcome.htm
19 *The Independent* (newspaper) 2 January 1996 p. 5 col. 1
20 Bero L A, Galbraith A, Rennie D. The publication of sponsored symposiums in medical journals. New England Journal of Medicine 1992 327 (16):1140–1153
21 Wald, N J et al Antenatal maternal serum screening for Down's syndrome: results of a demonstration project. British Medical Journal 1992 305 00: 391–394
22 CRD commentary for record 957089. University of York
23 http://wings.buffalo.edu/contest/awards/prof.html
24 http://www.gii-awards.com/nicampgn/3576.htm
25 http://cancer.med.upenn.edu/disease/testicular/tse.html
26 http://text.nlm.nih.gov/cps/www/cpsa10.html#Head.101
27 http://www/tcom.ohiou.edu/family-health/testicular-cancer.au
28 Journal of the American Medical Association 24/31 August 1994 p.645
29 http://wwwindex.nlm.nih.gov/publications/factsheets/online_databases.html
30 http://www.carl.org/uncover/updates/up195.html
31 http://www.who.ch/programmes/emc/flu/country.html

5

Interactive learning

Box 5.1 Chapter objectives

- Examine how medical education is being delivered over the Internet.
- Provide detailed descriptions of innovative examples of medical education on the Internet.
- Highlight the benefits of using the Internet for medical education.

INTRODUCTION

Though the Internet was originally devised for military and defence purposes, it was not long before academics, realising its potential, seized the initiative. Spurred on by a vision of the future where communication would be quick and simple (e-mail), and where research findings and data could be transferred at the touch of a button (FTP), the academic community began to invest time and money in developing computer networks.

As early as 1979, parts of the UK academic community were linked by a network created by the Science Research Council (SRC) and the National Education Research Council (NERC). By 1984, this network had expanded – and been renamed JANET (Joint Academic Network) – to enable *all* Universities and research laboratories to enjoy the benefits of wide area networking.

Throughout the late 1980s JANET continued to expand as more Polytechnics and Colleges of Higher Education sought access. In 1991, the JANET IPS (Internet protocol service) was created. This development meant that everyone on the JANET network could now access all the other computers on the Internet. By the same token, doctors and other health professionals who were not employed by a University department (or teaching hospital) could, for the first time, access the resources available on JANET. Though at the time this decision was not greeted with unbridled enthusiasm – indeed the only resources that were immediately available were University library catalogues – in retrospect it can be seen as a milestone in the development and use of the Internet in the UK.

As networks have grown and become more robust, academics and other professionals have begun to appreciate how they can be used in the process of teaching and learning. This chapter examines this development with reference to medical education on the Internet. Specifically, we will look at how the Internet is being used as a medium for delivering:

- virtual interactive consultations;
- medical tutorials and multimedia textbooks;
- interactive on-line courses;
- examinations;
- virtual conferencing.

For each of these subject areas one *innovative* Internet site will be discussed and assessed. For those who wish to explore further, other sites are recommended.

VIRTUAL INTERACTIVE CONSULTATIONS

From a patient's perspective, the most important skill a doctor should possess is the ability to diagnose illnesses quickly and accurately. Such a talent, however, tends to be acquired with practice and experience rather than theoretical learning. Indeed, it is highly probable that a recently qualified doctor will have had little direct contact with 'live' patients.

In recognition of this problem, a number of doctor/patient simulated encounters can now be experienced on the Internet. The best of these are described below.

The Interactive Patient

http://medicus.marshall.edu/medicus.htm

Developed by the Marshall University School of Medicine, *The Interactive Patient* is an inter-

active, World Wide Web program that allows you to simulate an actual patient consultation. The program begins by presenting the user with an opportunity to take a patient history. Information acquired here can be enhanced with a physical examination and by examining a range of laboratory results and X-rays. When a complete picture of the illness has been constructed, you are invited to submit a diagnosis and course of treatment.

What makes this product unique is the way you can directly *interact* with the patient. Thus, from the opening screen where the patient informs you of a 'pain in his side', the direction the interview takes is entirely under your control. For example, when asked the question 'Do you feel nauseous?', the patient replies,

Ever since the pain started at 9.00 a.m. this morning I have been somewhat nauseous. When the pain gets worse I start to feel sick in my stomach as well.

Using this answer as a clue to the nature of the illness, you can ask a follow-up question such as, 'Have you had any difficulty passing urine?' This questioning continues until you are satisfied that no further relevant information can be gleaned from the patient (Figs 5.1, 5.2).

If you ask a question that the patient is unable to answer, you are asked to be more specific; this simply means that the question does not contain any keywords that are present in *The Interactive Patient's* database.

As it is believed that around 82% of all out-patient diagnoses are based *exclusively* on what is learnt during the history-taking session, it is essential that considerable time should be spent on teaching students how to take full and accurate histories.[1] *The Interactive Patient* goes some way towards addressing this issue.

Once the history has been taken, you then have the opportunity to undertake a physical examination. Options currently available allow you to inspect, palpate or auscultate the patient. If you auscultate the heart (by pointing and clicking your mouse on the appropriate part of the patient's torso), you can

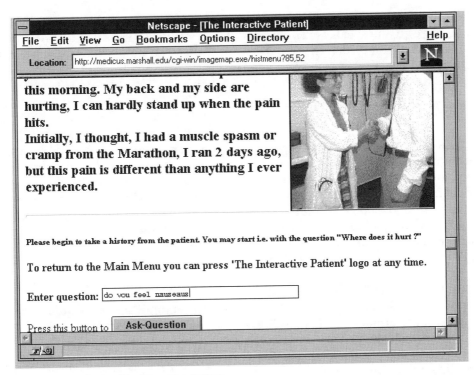

Fig. 5.1   Interviewing *The Interactive Patient*

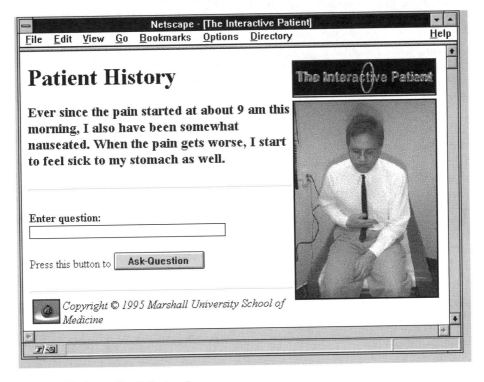

Fig. 5.2   *The Interactive Patient replies.*

actually hear how it sounds. If you do not have a sound card and speakers in your computer to support this function the sound will be described to you. In this example, the following message was relayed:

The heart sounds are regular without murmur. There is a prominent split S2.

The final pieces of the diagnosis jigsaw are the laboratory results and X-rays. More than 20 laboratory tests have been performed on this patient, ranging from vital signs (temperature, heart rate and blood pressure) to a complete blood count, and coagulation studies. For additional clues to the cause of the patient's pain, five radiological investigations have been performed. These include a chest X-ray, a CT scan of the lumbar vertebrae and an abdominal ultrasound.

Laden with this armoury of diagnostic evidence, you are finally invited to submit a diagnosis and indicate which of the suggested therapeutic options would be most effective. Depending on how busy the Marshall server is, a comment on your diagnosis and treatment is normally mailed to you within the hour.

Once you have successfully completed a case at the *Interactive Patient*, you will receive an electronic message containing an application form for a CME (Continuing Medical Education) Credit Certificate. A CME credit of 1 hour in 'Category 1 of the Physicians Recognition Award of the American Medical Association' is awarded for completing a case.[2]

With the imminent implementation of CME for all consultant staff in the UK, it can be anticipated (or hoped) that UK Web sites will also seek the right to award CME credits.[3]

Recommended sites for further exploration

University of Colorado Medical Rounds

http://www.uchsc.edu/sm/pmb/
medrounds/index.html

On accessing this page, you are presented with a history of the patient, a series of labora-

tory results, and the outcome of a physical examination. Unlike The *Interactive Patient*, there is no option for immediate interaction with the client to acquire additional information.

What you can do, however, is discuss specific aspects of the case with other health professionals who act as moderators. Via e-mail, you can submit questions or propose suggestions. After a week or so the pertinent parts of the patient's history that have not come to light through the questioning process, are disclosed along with a diagnosis and treatment plan. At this juncture, a new discussion forum is introduced.

Short Rounds Online – Stanford University

http://summit.stanford.edu/html/
consortium/srdc/demoSR.html

Like the Marshall and Colorado sites, physicians accessing the Stanford server are presented with information relating to the history of some anonymous patient, along with the results of a physical examination. Once sufficient information has been extracted from these sources, you are invited to diagnose the condition from a defined list. Should you misdiagnose, an explanation of *why* this cannot be correct is presented. In an educational context, this positive approach to error is more effective than the alternative, where you are simply informed that your diagnosis is incorrect.

MEDICAL TUTORIALS AND TEXTBOOKS

As more and more material relating to medical education is published on the Internet, traditional learning patterns and practices are being swept away. For example, in pre-Internet days if a medical student missed a lecture, the only option for the conscientious student was to copy up the notes from a colleague. Nowadays, it is possible that the lecture notes will be published on the Internet where they can be perused at a more convenient time.

Similarly, a student who wishes to supplement the lecture with some additional reading he is no longer constrained by the restrictive opening hours of the local medical library. Via the Internet, various medical textbooks and journals are available. Most strikingly, some of these will be multimedia publications enabling, for example, the student to hear abnormal lung sounds or watch a video of a surgical procedure.

Discussed below are some of the best examples on the Internet of this type of material.

Online Course in Medical Bacteriology

http://www.qmw.ac.uk/~rhbm001/intro.html

This on-line, read-only hypertext course on medical microbiology is aimed primarily at medical students who seek an introduction to this subject. Prepared by Dr Mark Pallen, Senior Lecturer in medical microbiology at St Bartholomew's Hospital Medical School in London, the course is split into seven modules covering topics such as 'The nature of bacteria' and 'The diagnosis of bacterial infections'.

On selecting the link to module 2, 'Bacteria in sickness and health', you are presented with a number of hypertext links. For example, you can read about natural flora in various parts of the body, learn how to judge whether or not a given bacterium is the cause of the given disease, or study definitions of some clinical syndromes caused by bacteria.

From the start of this tutorial, it is apparent that a great deal of care has gone into the development of these Web pages. To enable a student to follow the course sequentially – rather than jumping to specific links – the author has created 'next page' buttons. Similarly, recognising the importance of graphics to support and re-enforce the text, virtually every page contains 'high-impact diagrams'[4] as demonstrated in Figure 5.3.

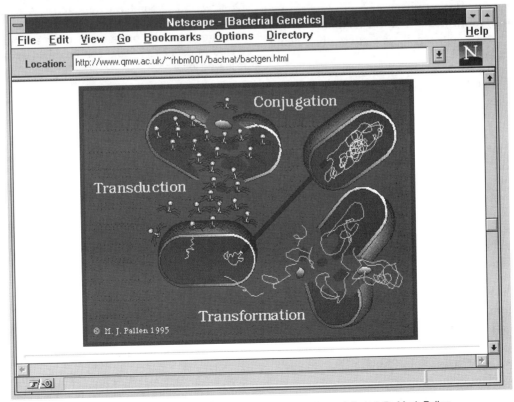

Fig. 5.3 High-impact diagram from the *Online Course in Medical Bacteriology* © Dr Mark Pallen

As an alternative to following the hypertext course, it is possible to FTP the lecture handouts. Note, however, that these are currently *only* available in an Apple Macintosh format.

The Virtual Hospital

Pediatric Airway Diseases: a multimedia textbook

The Virtual Hospital Home Page
http://vh.radiology.uiowa.edu/

example of a multimedia textbook
**http://indy.radiology.uiowa.edu/Providers/
Textbooks/peds/books/ElectricAirway/
ElectricAirway.html**

The Virtual Hospital defines itself as a 'continually updated digital health sciences library' providing information to both patients and health care providers 24 hours a day.[5] With regard to health care providers, the Virtual Hospital identifies the need to provide distance-learning facilities as one of its primary objectives. The provision of high-quality, up-to-date, multimedia medical textbooks is one way this objective is currently being addressed.

Twelve such texts, commissioned by the Virtual Hospital, are now available from this site. Topics covered range from muscle and back injuries, through to pulmonary embolus and gastrointestinal nuclear medicine. For illustrative purposes this section will examine just one book, *Pediatric Airway Diseases*.

Though the introductory page, with its table of contents, gives the appearance of an ordinary print-based textbook, as soon as you follow a hypertext link the true multimedia format of this book becomes apparent. For example, sprinkled within the text in the chapter on acute epiglottitis are numerous multimedia links that enable you to view and/or listen to:

- 7 videos that include how to observe and assess a child with epiglottitis without causing distress to the patient, and how to initiate mechanical ventilation;
- 6 still images that include an image of the

virus *Haemophilus influenza* type b, and an endolateral neck X-rays that shows classic swelling of the epiglottis;

- 1 sound clip to illustrate the stridorous sound of children who present with acute epiglottitis.

Even the text, which describes the nature of the illness and how it can be treated, has additional hypertext links to summary and discussion sections (Fig. 5.4).

To reinforce its purpose as a teaching tool, each chapter ends with a series of questions based on what you have read, listened to and watched. Mouse clicking on the 'Answer' hypertext link reveals the depth of your knowledge or ignorance.

Though the tag 'multimedia' seems to be appended to almost every publication on the Internet, those at the Virtual Hospital are some of the best examples of this format you are likely to encounter.

Note In common with most US Internet sites, the preferred software for displaying moving images is *Quicktime*. If you have an Apple Macintosh computer, then it is highly probable that this software is already present on your machine. For Windows users *Quicktime* can be FTPd from the following location:

ftp://ftp.support.apple.com

Recommended sites for further exploration

The Virtual Medical Centre

**http://www-sci.lib.uci.edu/~martindale/
Medical.html**

From this one point you can access a staggering 15 700 multimedia medical teaching files and modules, 23 200 multimedia medical courses, 173 multimedia medical school courses/textbooks, and 3500 video clips.

The Multimedia Medical Reference Library

http://www.tiac.net/users/jtward/index.html

This goes under the appellation of *Jonathan Tward's Multimedia Medical Reference Library* (Fig. 5.5).

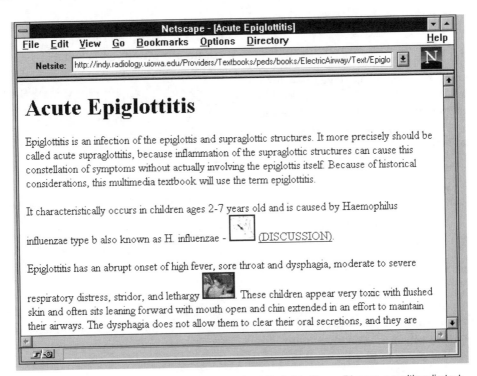

Fig. 5.4 Part of the chapter on acute epiglottitis from *Pediatric Airway Disease*, a multimedia textbook © University of Iowa: mouse-clicking on any 'thumbnail' image results in that image being magnified to full screen size

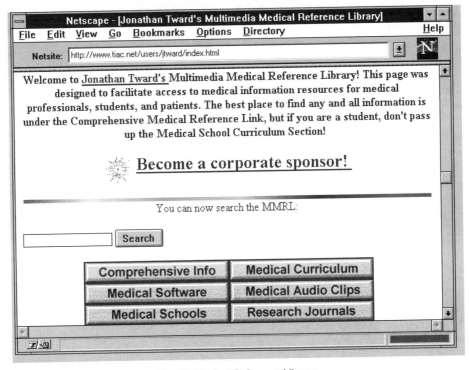

Fig. 5.5 *Jonathan Tward's Multimedia Medical Reference Library*

INTERACTIVE ON-LINE COURSES

For those students who require more than a read-only hypertext tutorial, interactive on-line courses are now being developed for the Internet.

One such course that may be of interest to the medical community is the *Online Course in Sequence Analysis*.

On-line Course in Sequence Analysis

http://www.techfak.uni-bielefeld.de/bcd/
   original-welcome.html

The course is also <u>mirrored</u> to a server at Manchester University. UK users should use this site for faster access:

http://info.mcc.ac.uk/hpctec/courses/
   Biocomputing/vsns/bcd/welcome.html

Run by the Virtual School of Natural Sciences, this 10-week course offers students a 'profound introduction to biosequence analysis and comparison'.[6]

Though the entire course is conducted over the Internet – thereby enabling you to follow it from your own home – in all other respects it takes the same format as any course you would attend at a university or college (Fig. 5.6). Thus, students are required to participate in discussion forums, work in groups and undertake individually assigned coursework. Completed assignments are transmitted for marking and comment by e-mail, whilst discussion and group work is facilitated by the virtual meeting place, <u>BioMOO</u> (see below).

When this course was first run in the summer of 1995, it attracted students and speakers from all parts of the world. Plans are now in hand to recruit students for the 1996 course.

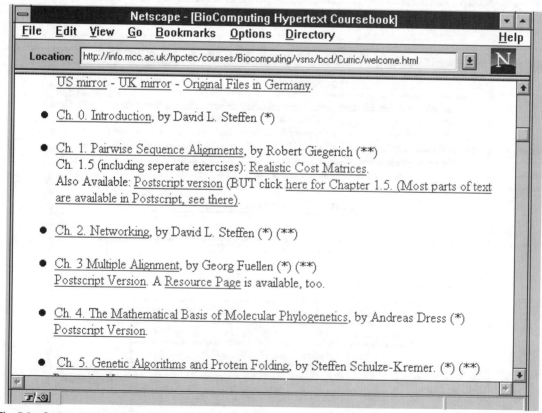

Fig. 5.6 Outline of the *Online Course in Sequence Analysis*

Recommended sites for further exploration

Principles of Protein Structure – Birkbeck College

http://www.cryst.bbk.ac.uk/PPS2/

Birkbeck College at the University of London, runs an Advanced Certificate course *Principles of Protein Structure,* via the Internet. As on the sequence analysis course, work assignments, self-assessment exercises and tutorials are conducted through e-mail and virtual reality discussion forums, such as BioMOO.

The cost of this 1-year course is £186.00 for students resident in the European Community, and £500.00 for anyone else (1996 prices). This course also serves as a timely reminder of how the Internet is becoming increasingly commercialised; when it was first run in 1995, no charges were levied.

ON-LINE EXAMINATIONS

A look at the loan statistics from any medical library will show conclusively that the items most frequently borrowed by medical staff are those which help them prepare for medical examinations. In the UK, this means books that focus on the Part I and Part II Membership and Fellowship examinations organised by the various Royal Colleges.

Though, as mentioned before, not one of the UK Royal Colleges has ventured onto the Internet, other bodies are taking the lead in developing computer assisted learning tools. MedWeb, at Birmingham University, is a good example of this.

MedWeb

http://medweb.bham.ac.uk/teaching.html

Recognising the need for medics to practice answering examination questions, staff at Birmingham University have developed a computer-assisted assessment facility that can be accessed over the Internet.

In its most basic form, the MedWeb server can be used to read and then answer a series of examination-type questions. When you have completed a test, you mouse click the 'Mark' button, and within a few minutes the results are e-mailed to you.

To simulate the different *types* of question you may encounter in an examination, MedWeb provides the opportunity to carry out MCQs, the more structured modified-essay questions, and short case studies. Figures 5.7 and 5.8 illustrate some of these different formats.

It is also possible to build your own test by instructing the MedWeb server to find only those questions that match your interest. For example, if you felt that you needed to practice answering questions that relate to the cardiovascular system, you can undertake a search of the Computer Assisted Assessment Database and retrieve only those questions that contain these keywords.

The *MedWeb* project is still very much in its infancy. Its long-term success depends on whether or not it can create a large enough MCQ/case study database to meet the disparate needs of the medical community. In recognition of this, users of the system are encouraged to submit their own questions and case studies.

Though commercialisation of the Internet is increasing, *MedWeb's* 'call for assistance' from its users typifies the spirit of cooperation and collaboration that ensures that the majority of Internet services are, and will continue to be, available without charge.

Recommended sites for further exploration

United Medical and Dental Schools Radiology (UMDS) Teaching File

http://www-ipg.umds.ac.uk/~acd/
index.htm

Though this site aims to provide educational material for *all* radiologists in training, the initial focus has been to help those candidates preparing for the Fellow of the Royal College of Radiologists (FRCR) Part I examination. A set of MCQs appropriate to this examination

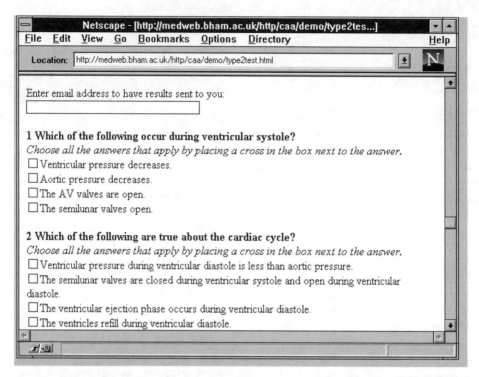

Fig. 5.7 MCQs at MedWeb

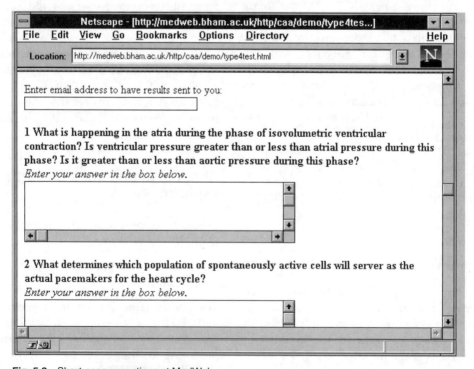

Fig. 5.8 Short-essay questions at MedWeb

are available for candidates to practice on, as are a series of radiological case studies (Fig. 5.9).

The healthy rivalry that exists between medical schools in the UK should result in a proliferation of teaching tools, similar to those developed by UMDS.

VIRTUAL CONFERENCING

A study conducted in 1988 on continuing education for general practitioners,[7] found that the main reasons for attending continuing education meetings were:

- they provided new information and reminders of things that were already known;
- they provided a useful means of meeting other general practitioners and consultants and, thus, provided a forum where common problems could be discussed.

In contrast, reasons for non-attendance included:

- lack of time;
- inconvenient meeting time;
- venue too far away.

Though in more recent years the GP contract, with its concomitant educational allowance, has added a financial incentive for attending educational meetings, the reasons identified for non-attendance are still valid.

However, using the internet it is now possible to enjoy the benefits of peer discussion and analysis *without* the trouble of attending some distant postgraduate centre. This dream-like scenario is made possible by the 'virtual conference' where physical attendance at a meeting is replaced by a virtual presence through your computer. BioMOO is the best example, at the moment, of a virtual meeting place.

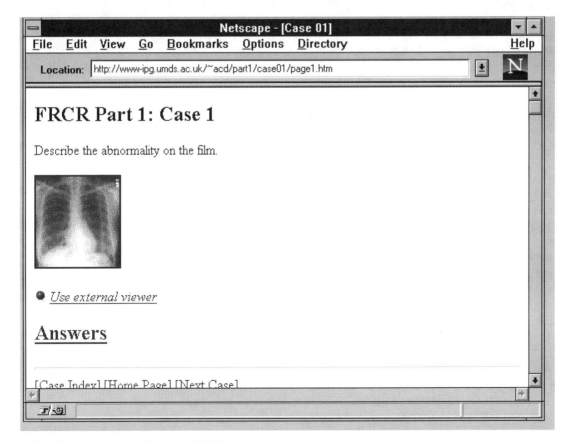

Fig. 5.9 Radiological case study from UMDS

In a similar vein the M.D. Anderson Cancer Center in the United States has started to use the Internet as a medium for transmitting live television teleconferences.

BioMOO

telnet://bioinfo.weizmann.ac.il: 8888
http://bioinformatics.weizmann.ac.il/
  BioMOO/

BioMOO is a text and image-based virtual reality system for all members of the international biology community. It is a place to meet colleagues studying biology and related disciplines, and an arena for hosting colloquia and conferences. The on-line course on sequence analysis for example, plans to hold its tutorials via BioMOO ('Interactive On-line Courses' above).

At BioMOO you can converse, in real time, with anyone else who is currently logged on. The medium for this is your computer keyboard and your Telnet client software. If a group of people arrange to log on to BioMOO at the same time, they can hold a meeting just as they would if they had booked a conference venue. The advantage of this method is that colleagues from around the world can attend without having the bother of getting to the location or finding accommodation.

In addition to being able to converse with colleagues, BioMOO also supports multimedia applications. Thus, it is possible to give a presentation, complete with full-colour slides and moving images, at a BioMOO conference just as you would at any 'real' conference or meeting. Users who wish to attend such a presentation, log on to BioMOO through their Telnet client and then, in parallel, open up a World Wide Web session. Specific instructions on how to do this are detailed in Box 5.2.

Once your log-on has been accepted, you will be presented with a series of hypertext links that allow you to see who else is currently logged on and what objects are available in that room (graphics, files, maps etc.). Figures 5.10, 5.11 and 5.12 show the BioMOO Lounge, Café, and Library and the objects they contain.

To move to another room you simply click on the mouse-sensitive map. To converse with anyone in the room switch to your Telnet window and type in your question, or comment.

Though BioMOO does not require users to wear virtual reality helmets and gloves, it is nevertheless a virtual world. The rooms you meet in only exist as concepts, and though at any point it may feel as if you are conversing with a group of people in one location, in reality the 'delegates' are likely to be scattered throughout the world.

Because MOOs (multiple user dimension object orientated) were originally devised as a computerised version of the adventure game *Dungeons and Dragons*, some people are still reluctant to concede their usefulness in a teaching environment. Any reader who questions the usefulness of BioMOO, however, should consider where else they could converse with colleagues from around the world, in a conference-like environment for the price of a local telephone call.

Box 5.2 Logging on to BioMOO

1   Using your Telnet client, log on to:
    bioinfo.weizmann.ac.il:8888

2   To log on as a guest, use the form:
    Prompt: *guest name password* (For example, guest rjk testing).

3   Resize the Telnet window so that you can see about five lines of text. Move this window to the bottom of the screen.

4   Load up your Web browser. Adjust the size of the window so that it sits above your Telnet window. Open location:
    http://bioinformatics.weizmann.ac.il/BioMOO/

5   Select the hypertext link 'Look into BioMOO'.

6   Select 'Web authentication system.' Use your BioMOO character name and password if you have a registered character, or the name and password you gave when connecting as a guest (for example, Log-in Name: *rjk* Password: *testing*).

7   Welcome to the BioMOO Lounge.

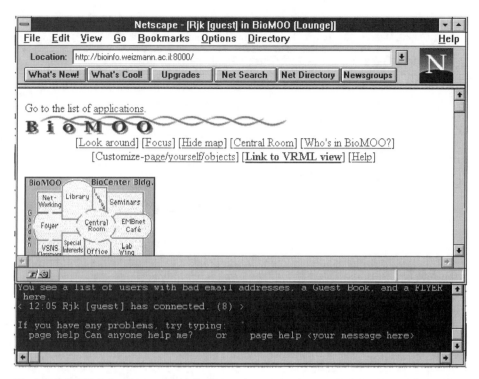

Fig. 5.10 BioMOO: the Telnet window at the bottom of the screen is used to communicate with other delegates whilst the Web window is used to view multimedia applications

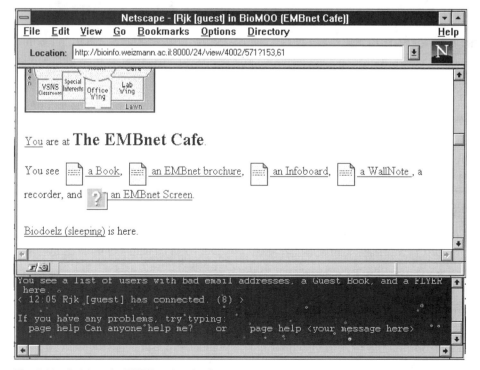

Fig. 5.11 A visit to the EMBNet virtual cafe

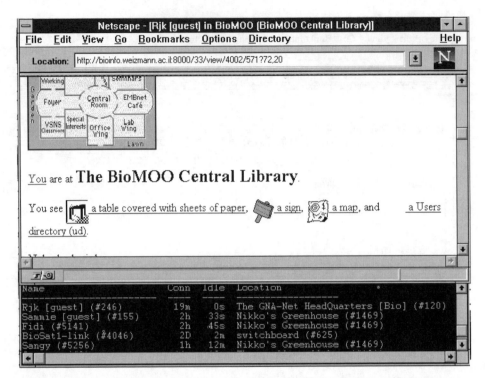

Fig. 5.12 The BioMOO Library: the Telnet window is displaying who else is currently logged on – to see this type *who* in your Telnet window

Video conferencing

M. D. Anderson Cancer Center: University of Texas

http://utmdacc.mda.uth.tmc.edu/

Another approach to the virtual meeting has been adopted by the M. D. Anderson Cancer Center, at the University of Texas. Aware that primary care physicians in rural parts of Texas are unwilling to travel long distances to attend continuing education meetings, the Anderson Cancer Center has started to transmit live lectures over the Internet using Cornell University's video conferencing program, *CU-SeeMe* (pronounced 'see you see me').

The first lecture on breast cancer, transmitted in April 1995, was routed to a CU-SeeMe reflector which meant that any Internet user who had a copy of the *CU-SeeMe* client software could view this teleconference (Fig. 5.13). Plans are currently in hand to re-broadcast

this and deliver other teleconferences on prostate, cervical, and colonic cancer.

CU-SeeMe allows you to see, hear and speak with others, in real time, via the Internet. *CU-SeeMe* supports both one-to-one, and one-to-many video conferencing. To facilitate the latter, the organisation (or person) transmitting the teleconference needs to route it via a CU-SeeMe reflector, which acts like a mini television station. In the United States, there are a number of public reflectors that, subject to the rules of 'netiquette', anyone can use.

Perhaps the most exciting thing about *CU-SeeMe* is that it works over low-speed modem links. Though 28 800 bps is the preferred minimum speed, users have reported that conferences are viewable – if a little jerky – at 14 400 bps. Moreover, it is also a very cheap way to watch or broadcast a conference. Both the client and reflector software for the PC and Apple Macintosh can be FTPd without charge from Cornell University,[8] whilst the only hard-

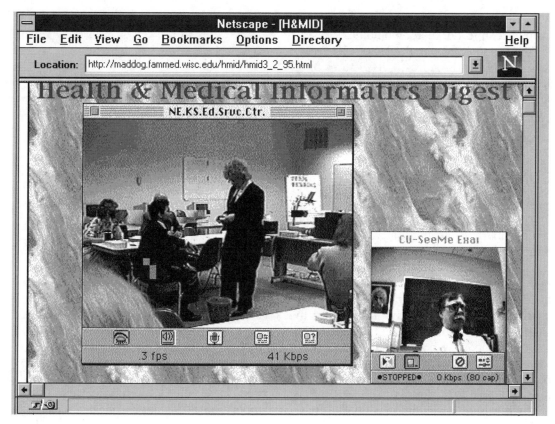

Fig. 5.13 Pictures of the *CU-SeeMe* teleconference transmitted by the M. D. Anderson Cancer Center, captured by *Health & Medical Informatics Digest*
http: //maddog.fammed.wisc.edu/hmid/hmid3_2_95.html

ware you need to broadcast a conference is a camcorder. (An article published in the magazine *Urban Desires* recently reported that a black-and-white digital camcorder can be acquired for less than US $100.00).[9]

If you would like to know more about video conferencing using *CU-SeeMe* point your Web browser at:

**ftp://gated.cornell.edu/pub/video/html/
  Welcome.html**

Recommended sites for further exploration

GenomeMOO

Health professionals with a specific interest in genome information will find the GenomeMOO

a valuable source of information. This MOO can be accessed at:

telnet://straylight.tamu.edu:7777

More CU-SeeMe uses

For another practical illustration of *CU-SeeMe* being used in an educational context, point your Web browser at the following location:

**http://kmi.open.ac.uk/kmi-misc/
  virtualsummer.html**

Here you will find a discussion of how the Open University in the UK used *CU-SeeMe* technology to run a 'virtual summer school'. Using this software students following the undergraduate course in cognitive psychology were able to participate in group discussions, obtain one-to-one tutorials, listen to and watch lectures, and work in project teams – all from the comfort of their own homes.

For a non-educational use of *CU-SeeMe*, note that NASA broadcast live pictures of all space shuttle launches on the Internet via this software. For more details see:

**http://btree.lerc.nasa.gov/NASA_TV/
NASA_TV.html**

CONCLUSION

As a health sciences librarian, one of my primary responsibilities is to introduce health professionals to the Internet. This is usually done through a hands-on tour of some key medical sites, including many of the ones highlighted in this chapter. In doing this, the overriding impression I am left with is how much enjoyment they derive from using the Internet. This is not surprising. Indeed, there can be few people who are not attracted by the idea of multimedia textbooks, simulated patient consultations, and meetings conducted in Virtual Reality.

Apart from making the process of studying and learning more enjoyable, using the Internet as a medium for delivering medical education has other advantages, which are summarised in Box 5.3.

Box 5.3 Using the Internet for medical education: key benefits

- You can study at a time that is convenient to you.
- You do not have to travel to participate in a conference or meeting – but can still enjoy the benefits of live, interactive discussion.
- As virtual meetings attract colleagues and experts form around the world, it can be assumed that the discussion will be more informed than that which occurs at a local meeting.
- Delivering a virtual conference can be done from your own home or place of work thereby saving time and expense. Funds that would have been consumed on travel and accommodation can now be diverted to patient care.
- Sate-of-the-art multimedia teaching tools and textbooks are available 24 hours a day.

Though I do not believe the Internet will replace the library or the Postgraduate Medical Centre, it will provide additional opportunities for health professionals to further their medical education. In the longer term, this will create a better qualified workforce that, in turn, can deliver patient care more effectively.

REFERENCES AND NOTES

1 Hampton R et al Relative contributions of history-taking, physical examination and laboratory investigation to diagnosis and management of medical outpatients. British Medical Journal 1975 2:486–489

2 http://medicus.marshall.edu/cme.htm

3 Royal College of Physicians of the United Kingdom Recommendations for the introduction and implementation of a CME system. RCP 1994

4 http://www.qmw.ac.uk/~rhbm001/intro.html

5 http://vh.radiology.uiowa.edu/Welcome/About VH.html

6 http://info.mcc.ac.uk/hpctec/courses/ Biocomputing/vsns/bcd/welcome.html

7 Alan Branthwaite et al Continuing education for General Practitioners. Royal College of General Practitioners 1988 (Occasional Paper 38)

8 ftp://gated.cornell.edu/pub/video/html/ Welcome.html

9 Meloan S Tech-Toys: Cu-SeeMe. Urban Desires at: http://desires.com/1.6/Toys/Cuseeme/cuseeme.html

6

E-mail, discussion lists and newsgroups

Box 6.1   Chapter objectives

- Introduce and discuss e-mail, discussion lists and newsgroups; three of the most useful services available on the Internet.

- Explain the function of these, and demonstrate with practical examples their value to health professionals.

- Highlight potential problems and concerns – such as the security of e-mail, or the relevance of newsgroup postings – and suggest ways in which these can be resolved.

INTRODUCTION

For many people, the catalyst for getting connected to the Internet is the wish (or need) to be able to send and receive e-mail. Indeed, despite the attention that is afforded to applications like the World Wide Web, and this book is no exception to this, e-mail is still the most widely used service on the Internet.

In addition to being able to communicate with friends and colleagues, e-mail is also the method used for contributing to discussion lists and newsgroups. This chapter looks at these services, and focuses on how they can help health professionals in their day-to-day work. To begin though, it is necessary to have an understanding of what e-mail is, and why it is so important.

E-MAIL

Defined simply, e-mail is a method for transferring information from one location to another. This information can be in the form of a text file or, as is increasingly common, a binary file. Examples of the latter type include word-processed documents, spreadsheets or graphics. For completeness it should be noted that e-mail can also be used to retrieve World Wide Web pages and even files from FTP sites.[1]

Why use it?

To some, it might appear a curious paradox that users of the world's most advanced network of computers – the Internet – rely upon the traditional written word as their main method of communication. This situation does not reflect a wish to return to bygone days but the realisation that e-mail is the most effective method of communication that has yet been devised. Compared with traditional mail, known by Internet aficionados as 'snail mail', e-mail has many advantages. In particular, for the reasons listed in Box 6.2, it is quick, cheap and efficient.

Compared to the other electronic communication media, telephone and fax, e-mail again scores well. For example, if you wish to communicate with a number of colleagues – some of whom may be overseas – both the fax and phone will prove expensive. In addition to this, neither medium can handle binary files, and the chances of the message reaching the intended recipient depend on unquantifiable variables such as whether or not the person is in (to answer the phone), and whether or not the fax machine is engaged, switched on or even loaded with sufficient paper. E-mail messages encounter none of these problems. Figure 6.1 illustrates how users who have a dial-up connection to the Internet send and receive e-mail.

The advantages highlighted in Box 6.2 apply to all users of e-mail, but there are other benefits that seem particularly pertinent to health professionals (Box 6.3).

Though undoubtedly e-mail is a 'good thing', there is one caveat that should not be overlooked: if you have a dial-up connection to the Internet, it is up to *you* to go and collect your mail. Though a message from the other side of the world may hit your mailbox within minutes of it being sent, if you do not routinely empty your mailbox (by dialling into your Internet provider) this significant advantage is lost.

It is also worth pointing out that most Internet providers will only hold mail for a certain period. Demon Internet, for example, will hold mail for up to 30 days. After this time, any mail that has not been collected is returned to the sender.

Box 6.2 The main advantages of e-mail

Speed
Exactly how long a message takes to get from A to B depends on factors such as network traffic, and how many individual networks a particular message has to go through. Experts agree, however, that *most* messages are delivered in 2–3 hours, and it is not unusual for a message to land in someone's mail box seconds after it has been sent.

Cost
It costs no more to send a message from London to Australia than it does from London to Oxford. And, though a large file may entail a slightly longer connection to your Internet provider, these costs will be negligible when compared to the cost of airmailing or sending the same document by courier.

Efficiency
Assuming you have addressed your message correctly, then for the most part, your mail will get delivered. On occasions when this is not possible – the recipient is no longer 'in residence' for example – your mail will be returned. In Internet parlance, mail is 'bounced'.

Box 6.3 The benefits of e-mail for health professionals

- A scan through the contents of any current medical journal reveals how many articles are co-authored. Using e-mail, it is easy to circulate drafts of a paper to all authors who can comment, and then add their contribution, without ever having to re-key any text.

- If you encounter a rare medical condition and require guidance on how it should be managed, you can solicit expert opinion from around the world with just one e-mail message. Further details are given in 'Discussion lists' and 'Newsgroups' (below).

- Because the collection of mail is done at a time that is convenient to you, interruptions to your day can be minimised.

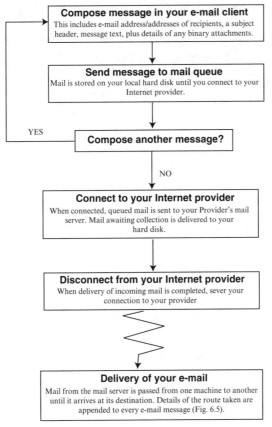

Fig. 6.1   Sending and receiving e-mail: a schematic overview

---

Box 6.4   Core features required in an e-mail client

Text editing features
These allow you to cut and paste text.

'Reply' and 'Forward' options
Another factor that has contributed to the popularity of e-mail is the ease with which replies can be generated. On hitting the 'Reply' button, the mail software automatically creates a new message with the addressee details already completed. The original message may also be copied to this file to facilitate the composition of comments and answers (see below). Forwarding mail to other colleagues is achieved with the 'Forward' function.

Easy addressing facilities
As e-mail addresses tend be long and instantly forgettable, it is important that your mail client has an address book function in which frequently used e-mail addresses can be stored and accessed. If you have a list

of users to whom you mail regularly, then the option to create a distribution list is also useful.

'Confirmation of Delivery' option
When you use this option, an automatic message is mailed to you confirming that your e-mail has reached the recipient's mailbox. Some mailers also allow you to receive confirmation that the message has been read. The days for claiming that the mail 'must have got lost in the post' are clearly numbered.

An option to attach binary files to your messages
A good mailer will allow you to simply press the 'Attach' button, and prompt you for the name of the file you wish to send. As binary files need to be packaged – encoded – in a particular way before they can be sent over the Internet, a mail client that can do this (and decode received binary files) is to be preferred. Clients that can perform these tasks are said to be MIME compliant.

E-mail clients

To be able to compose, send and read e-mail you must use either a dedicated e-mail <u>client</u>, or have a mail facility within your <u>Web browser</u> (Figs 6.2, 6.3). Your Internet provider

should supply you with an e-mail program; if not, or if you wish to change clients, refer back to 'Finding and FTPing Software' in Chapter 2.

Whatever mail client you use, it should support the core features described in Box 6.4.

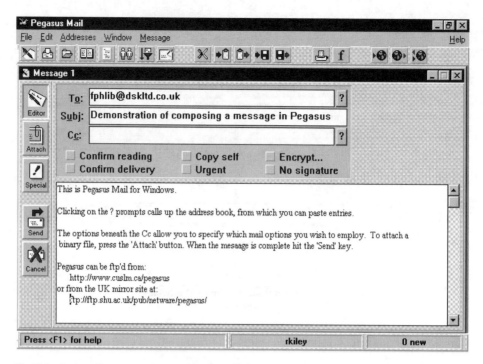

Fig. 6.2 Composing an e-mail message using *Pegasus* e-mail client for Windows

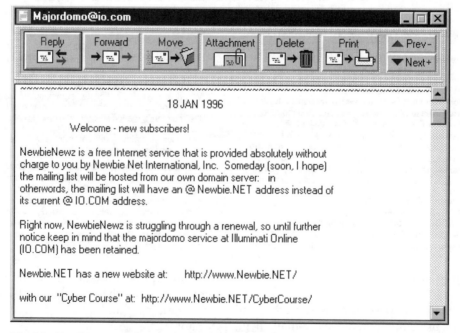

Fig. 6.3 Reading an e-mail message using *Pegasus* e-mail client for Windows. Note the push button approach to replying, forwarding and other options

```
Date sent:        Mon, 4 Dec 95 20: 44: 46 PST
From:             philip@ICSI.Net
Subject:          FW: Questions for a book
To:               rkiley@rkiley.demon.co.uk
Copies to:        tom@ICSI.Net

Dear Mr. Kiley:

Regarding your questions:

>>Specifically, can you search on trade name as well as drug name?

Yes, when you search for a name it searches both generic and brand names.

>>How much does this service cost?

Per year US$169, 6 month US$89.

>>Can you bill in sterling?

We can charge a credit card in US$.

Thanks for your interest in Physicians GenRx. If you have any other
questions, please feel free to direct them to me personally.
─────────────────────────────────────────
Philip Suarez, M.D.                 philip@icsi.net
─────────────────────────────────────────
           Physicians GenRx on the World Wide Web
        Medicine's most complete drug compendium resource
                  now available by subscription:
                    http://www.icsi.net/GenRx
```

Fig. 6.4 Using the 'Reply' function

The 'Reply' function

Figure 6.4 illustrates how this works. You should note that the return address was created automatically, and that the original message has been prefixed with >> symbols.

The header

Every e-mail message you send and receive is delivered in a 'virtual envelope', known as the header. Like its paper equivalent, this envelope contains details such as the name and address of the recipient, when it was posted, and who sent it. As a message passes through different networks on the Internet, additional franking data are appended to the header.

For the most part, you can let your mail client hide the header from view, but it can be useful for troubleshooting if things go wrong, or if you are simply curious to see how long a message took to reach you.

Figure 6.5 shows the route and the time it took for a message posted in Wisconsin to reach Demon Internet in London. Read the explanatory comments, shown in italics, from bottom to top.

Finding addresses

If you dial a telephone number incorrectly you either receive an 'unobtainable' tone or get connected to the wrong person. E-mail addresses work in much the same way in that incorrectly addressed mail is either 'bounced' or delivered to a complete stranger. However, whereas telephone users can rely on directory enquiry services to identify the correct number, e-mail users often have to resort to sleuthing and ingenuity.

The easiest way to obtain someone's e-mail address is to telephone them and ask. However, if this is impractical or inconvenient, there are some other methods you can employ. First, you can use one of the growing number of Internet White Page Services, such as Netfind or Four11. Four11, for example, is a database comprising more than 3 million e-mail addresses that can be searched by surname and/or Internet domain name. Though easy to use, the coverage is patchy; I was unable to find my e-mail address though other Demon Internet clients were listed.

A second approach is to search the Mailbase membership database (see below). Though only 60 000 e-mail addresses are stored here, the education and research focus of the Mailbase discussion lists means that the find rate for health professionals is relatively high.

To search this index point your Web browser at:

**http://www.mailbase.ac.uk/
search-names.html**

If you know *where* the person you are seeking is employed, a final approach is to see if the employing institution has a presence on the World Wide Web (Ch. 3). If it has a presence, then it is possible that the Web site will have a link to a staff index that can either be searched or browsed.

From rbrown@maddog.fammed.wisc.edu Tue, 2 Jan 96 11:30:44

E-mail from rbrown delivered to my local hard disk

X-Envelope-To: <rkiley@rkiley.demon.co.uk>

Delivery address

Return-Path: <rbrown@maddog.fammed.wisc.edu>

Reply address – this is how the 'Reply' function works

Received: from punt2.demon.co.uk by rkiley.demon.co.uk
id b494e762 Tue, 2 Jan 96 11:30:41

Collected by me from Demon Internet (my provider) on 2 January. By comparing this time with that displayed at the top of the header, we see that the transfer time from Demon Internet to my local hard disk was 3 seconds.

Received: from punt-2.mail.demon.net by mailstore for rkiley@rkiley.demon.co.uk
id 820253730:01454:0; Fri, 29 Dec 95 16:15:30 GMT

This message was placed in my mailbox on the 29 December 1995 at 16.15

Received: from relay-1.mail.demon.net ([158.152.1.140]) by punt-
2.mail.demon.net
id aa01200; 29 Dec 95 16:14 GMT
    Passed to second Demon mail server, called punt-2

Received: from maddog.fammed.wisc.edu ([144.92.222.220])
by relay-1.mail.demon.net id aa19346; 29 Dec 95 16:14 GMT

Received by Demon Internet mail server at 16.14 GMT on 29th December 95. As CST is 6 hours behind GMT, the total time this message took to get from Wisconsin to Demon Internet was 4 minutes.

Received: by maddog.fammed.wisc.edu;
id AA19436; 4.1/42; Fri, 29 Dec 95 10:10:48 CST

Message received by mail server at Wisconsin University at 10.10 CST

From: Roger Brown <rbrown@maddog.fammed.wisc.edu>

Full name and e-mail address of sender

Message-Id: <9512291010.AA19436@maddog.fammed.wisc.edu>

Every mail item has a unique identifier

Subject: Medical teleconferences

Subject of the e-mail

To: rkiley@rkiley.demon.co.uk

Addressee

Date: Fri, 29 Dec 95 10:10:48 CST

Date and time mail sent

X-Mailer: ELM [version 2.3 PL6]

Type and name of the e-mail client that was used

Fig. 6.5 The e-mail header: read from bottom to top

Security

Mail sent electronically is often likened to a postcard in that it can be read as it makes its way from sender to recipient. However, whereas a postman or sorting clerk will tire long before reading anything to their advantage, computer programs looking for 'trigger words' never will. Consequently, if you are going to use e-mail to send sensitive or confidential data, encryption is highly recommended.

In essence there are two kinds of encrypting technique. The first, made available by some mail clients, enables you to transform your mail into a random string of characters that can only be deciphered if the recipient knows the password. As sending the password by e-mail would negate the object of the exercise, the sender must find some other way of notifying the recipient of the correct password. As you can imagine, this is not particularly practical and is not widely used.

A second, and better method is based on public/private key encryption. Users of this encryption technique employ a piece of software to generate two alpha/numeric 'keys'. The private key, held on the users computer is never disclosed, whilst the public key is made available to everyone. Anyone can then use this public key to send an encrypted message to this person, but *only* the recipient, who has the second half of the key, can decrypt the message.

If you wish to use this form of encryption, a freeware program known as *Pretty Good Privacy* (*PGP*) can be FTPd from either of the following locations:

Non-US citizens:
http://www.ifi.uio/~staalesc/PGP/
US citizens:
http://web.mit.edu/network/pgp.html

The reason there are two sites is because it is illegal to export (or FTP) this software from the United States. The US State Department consider *PGP* to be strong cryptographic technology and as such regulate its export via the International Traffic in Arms Regulations (ITAR). But as long as you have FTPd *PGP* from the appropriate location, it is perfectly legal to use it.

The attempt by the US government to stop this technology falling into 'enemy' hands reflects the fact that it is virtually impossible to decipher *PGP* encrypted mail. An example of a *PGP* public key is shown in Figure 6.6.

Viruses

In recent months, there has been much talk in the press about computer viruses being transmitted by e-mail.[2] The most famous of these has been the winword.concept virus that disguises itself as a document template in a Microsoft *Word for Windows* file. When the recipient opens a mail item infected with this virus, another program is automatically launched. This second program executes a set of defined procedures, with potentially disastrous results.

Though Microsoft described this virus as a 'prank' they have been sufficiently concerned to release an antidote. If you use *Word for Windows*, and want to be sure that e-mail attachments that use this application are not infected, then FTP the following file:

http://www.microsoft.com/msoffice/freestuf/ msword/download/mvtool/mvtool2.exe

To keep this threat in proportion, one should remember that most messages received electronically are text files and as such must be virus-free. When a file is accompanied with a binary attachment, it is good practice to scan these files with an up-to-date virus checker before they are opened.

Conventions and netiquette

When conversing by telephone, our tone of voice adds meaning to what we are saying. Similarly when sending a letter by post we clarify the message in a variety of ways; job applications tend to be submitted on high quality vellum-like paper, whilst letters to a lover may be enclosed in a scented envelope, adorned with the acronym SWALK. The recip-

```
————BEGIN PGP PUBLIC KEY BLOCK————Version: 2.6.2i

mQCNAjCt8doAAAEEAMRXWcI/9GZbZK7esehTXGjYhHnadWJlEo7eXR+1dkkPcwNtSdJO3hIWL71mmSU
YmvWBfXV7iJ/Ek7ipb/TxATtUwCJtUvV/mWaTkcsNYiHtBU3T8Sz4R4eRF0BUa2YoCIWxJQng9FQa2MdT7
DHbHxckVPPKXcTHhRjJtTkrg+ilAAURtChMZXMgU21pdGhzb24gPGxzbWl0aHNvbkBhcmMuUuZGVtb24uY2
8udWs+tAxMZXMgU21pdGhzb24==yWge
————END PGP PUBLIC KEY BLOCK————
```

Fig. 6.6 A *PGP* public key

ient of a message sent electronically however, has to rely *exclusively* on the written word.

To minimise the risk of misunderstandings, e-mail users have devised various codes (known as smileys or emote-icons) that you can add to the text to clarify your meaning. For example, to indicate that you are joking you can append your comments with a :-) (read this sideways). Should you ever wish to indicate that you are a drunk, devilish chef with a toupee, a moustache and double chin, use the following:

C=}>; *{))

For more examples of this art :-), see the *Unofficial Smiley Dictionary* at:

http://manuel.brad.ac.uk/Network/
eegtti-2.3/eeg_286.html#SEC287

A good rule of thumb, however, is that if your message is likely to be misunderstood, rephrase it.

To minimise the amount of text you have to type and to keep messages concise, a number of e-mail acronyms have been adopted. IM(H)O 'in my (humble) opinion', BTW 'by the way' and TIA 'thanks in advance' are, perhaps, the most common, and the most useful.

Finally, good netiquette (etiquette on the Internet) dictates that:

- your messages should not be composed in CAPITAL LETTERS as it appears as if you are shouting;
- your e-mail signature should be no more than three lines long;
- mailings to a newsgroup or discussion list should be relevant and worthwhile. Re-posting someone else's message with the comment 'I agree' will not endear you to other Internet users.

ELECTRONIC DISCUSSION LISTS

Discussion lists (or mailing lists as they are sometimes called), are subject specific discussion groups that are participated in and distributed by e-mail. Once you have joined a list – for instance, research into drug misuse or medical infomatics – every message that is subsequently posted to that list is copied to your electronic mailbox. This task is per-formed by computer programs known as list-servers.

Mailing lists are an excellent way in which health professionals can seek opinion, air concerns, and discuss topics of mutual interest. For example, subscribers to the *Evidence-based health*[3] mailing list have, in the past few weeks, discussed the purpose of evidence-based medicine, the availability of MRI clinical guidelines, and have been kept informed of appropriate job vacancies (Fig. 6.7).

It should be noted that the *majority* of discussion lists are open to everyone. Though the discussion list *gp-uk*[4] – with its emphasis on education and training for general practitioners in the UK – will be of little interest to most people, there is nothing to stop *anyone* following the discussions or posting questions to the list.

In recognition of this, a number of moderated medical discussion lists have started to appear. For example, potential subscribers to *vascunet*[5] – the vascular surgery mailing list – have to demonstrate that they are medically qualified *before* they are admitted to the list. Though this means that someone has to manually vet potential subscribers, the end result should be a more informed, and thus more useful, discussion group.

Whatever the status of the list, all subscribers should remember how easy it is to forward e-mail to other people. A message you thought was going to a select and discreet group of people can be forwarded, at the touch of a button, to other lists and other people. With this in mind, you should never send anything by e-mail you would not want to become public knowledge.

Finding lists pertinent to your interests

If you total the number of mailing lists hosted by the four major listservers (Listserv, Listprocessor, Majordomo and Mailbase) you will discover that you have the option to subscribe to more than 13 000 discussion lists.

To identify which lists most closely match your interests either consult one of the indexing resources such as Medical Matrix or

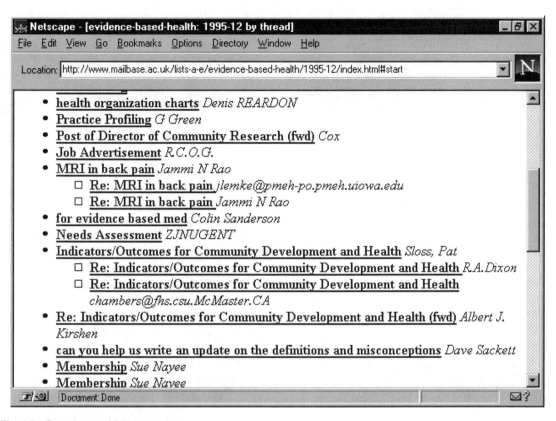

Fig. 6.7   Browsing the Mailbase archive

HealthWeb (Ch. 3), or search the listserver database at the following address:

http://www.liszt.com/

As this database only contains the *names* of the mailing lists and their one-line descriptions, you may have to try several searches to find what you're looking for. For example, searching on 'medicine' will not retrieve every medical-related mailing list in the database; you need to try more specific terms such as 'inflammatory bowel diseases', 'stroke' or 'neurosurgery'.

Though the coverage of this database is extensive, it does not index the Mailbase discussion lists. As these originate in the UK, and are only established if they can be seen to benefit the higher education and research community, they are particularly useful to health professionals practising in the UK. Names and

descriptions of Mailbase lists can be searched at:

http://www.mailbase.ac.uk/ search-descriptions.html.

Searching this database for the term 'health' identified 15 mailing lists including *public-health* – 'a discussion forum and information resource for those working in epidemiology and public health'[6] – and *nukop-health* a list that provides 'updates on health policy related UK government publications and a forum to discuss matters arising from them'.[7]

The Mailbase server also maintains an archive of all discussion list postings. Users can access this to assess the quality and relevance of a discussion list *before* subscribing. The fact that mailings are archived further reinforces the need to be circumspect when participating in group discussions.[8]

Joining, contributing to, and leaving a discussion list

To join a discussion list you simply send an e-mail to the listserver that hosts the list, indicating the name of the list you wish to subscribe to and your 'real' name. There is no need to include your e-mail address as this will be picked up automatically by the listserver. Figure 6.8 shows you how to join the list *gp-uk*.

To:	mailbase@mailbase.ac.uk
Subject:	*leave blank*
Text:	subscribe gp-uk *firstname surname*

Fig. 6.8 Joining discussion list *gp-uk*

An automatic acknowledgement of your subscription will be mailed to you, along with instructions on how to contribute to the list and how to leave the list.

It may sound somewhat trivial and pedantic, but perhaps the most important thing to learn about discussion lists is the difference between the address of the *mailing list* and the address of the *listserver*. All e-mail relating to the administration of the list (subscribing, suspending etc.) must be sent to the listserver, whilst contributions to the discussion are sent to the list. Whereas Figure 6.8 is addressed to the listserver, Figure 6.9 is addressed to the *gp-uk* mailing list. Every individual who subscribes to this list receives a copy of this message.

Once you have joined a discussion list, it is important to collect your e-mail on a regular basis. Contributing to a discussion that took place some time ago and has now moved on, will not endear you to the other list members.

You should also be aware that some discussion lists are *very* active. If you defer collecting your mail for a few days you may be surprised by the number of messages that have accumulated, and how long it takes to download and read them.

To:	gp-uk@mailbase.ac.uk
Subject:	Deputising Services
Text:	Our practice is considering introducing a deputising service for out of hours calls. Any comments on the effectiveness, costs, or problems that may result would be appreciated. I will summarise the findings for the list.

Fig. 6.9 Contributing to a discussion list. Note that offering to summarise the findings of such a request is considered to be good netiquette.

Similarly, if you are going to be away for a long time, check the documentation that was mailed with your subscription confirmation to see if the listserver supports 'suspend' and 'resume' functions.

Finally, netiquette and common sense dictate that all contributions should be relevant and, unless specifically permitted, you should not use a discussion list for advertising purposes.

USENET NEWS: NEWSGROUPS

Newsgroups are another way in which the Internet facilitates group communication. Arranged on a subject-specific basis, newsgroups enable groups of like-minded people to ask questions, raise concerns and discuss topics of mutual interest. For example, fans of the BBC Radio programme *The Archers* can read and contribute to the *uk.media.radio.archers* newsgroup, whilst aficionados of lotteries may find the *rec.gambling.lottery* newsgroup essential reading. Alternatively, health professionals with a special interest in cardiology or AIDS may care to follow the discussions in the *sci.med.cardiology* or *sci.med.aids* newsgroups.

Current estimates suggest that there are over 15 000 newsgroups, catering for every interest, speciality, and perversion known. The tabloid-generated myth that the Internet is merely a repository of pornography is, to a large degree, the consequence of a small minority of Internet newsgroups.

Though the purpose of newsgroups and discussion lists is the same – to share information on a group-wide basis – they differ in the following respects:

- postings to a newsgroup are held on a newsgroup server rather than copied to your personal electronic mailbox;

- you do not formally subscribe to a newsgroup.

Not subscribing means that if, on a particular day, you wish to read postings made to the *talk.politics.medicine* newsgroup you merely indicate this via your newsgroup client (see below). There is no newsgroup equivalent of the listserver.

Internet newsgroups attract huge international audiences and are, therefore, excellent arenas in which to solicit opinions and seek advice. For example, the newsgroup *news.newusers.questions* – set up as a forum for discussing issues and raising questions about Internet newsgroups – attracts a daily readership of 160 000 people.[9] Though the more specialised groups attract smaller audiences they are still fairly substantial. The *sci.med.aids*

Box 6.5 How to ensure you can participate in Usenet newsgroups

- Your Internet provider must have a 'news feed' service. Messages sent to newsgroups are propagated around the Internet by a protocol known as NNTP (network news transport protocol). If your provider does not have a NNTP server then you will not be able to participate in any newsgroup.[11]

- You must have a client on your computer that can interpret data sent from a NNTP server. Typically, this will take the form of a dedicated newsreader, or your Web browser if it has been 'news enabled'. (Newsgroups can be read through the *Netscape* Web browser (Appendix B).

---

newsgroup attracts 26 000 readers and even the highly specific *sci.med.telemedicine* newsgroup boasts a daily readership of around 14 000.[10] To participate in this globally distributed discussion system, you must have the facilities outlined in Box 6.5

The choice of newsreader client will depend upon your operating system and what is currently available. Whichever client you opt for, it should support:

- message 'threading' (Fig. 6.10);
- an off-line reading facility.

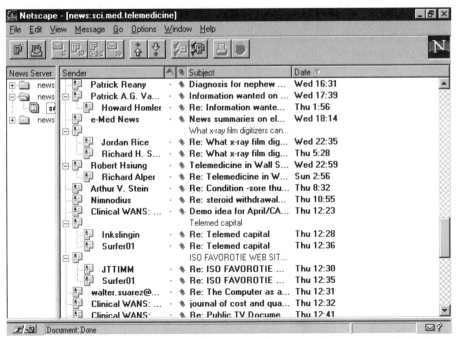

Fig. 6.10 Newsgroup messages through *Netscape*: replies to a posting are indented below the original message

Message threading sorts messages by the subject heading so that replies are shown next to the original message. Off-line reading is essential because almost all newsgroups attract large numbers of postings. It is, therefore, prudent to collect them from the NNTP server and read them once your connection to your Internet provider has been severed.

Arrangement of newsgroups

To help the user navigate his way through the mass of newsgroups, a hierarchical approach has been adopted. Table 6.1 shows the most important newsgroup categories, with examples to illustrate how the main category is further subdivided.

In addition to these category groups, you may also encounter newsgroups that are restricted to specific regions or organisations. Subscribers to Demon Internet for example, have access to a range of Demon newsgroups where problems, questions, and news specific to Demon users can be discussed.

Precisely which newsgroups are available to you is determined by your Internet provider. However, though some do not have a news feed to the *alt.sex* range of newsgroups, the majority of providers can be expected to carry the scientific range of newsgroups most sought after by health professionals.

Finding relevant newsgroups

With so many newsgroups available, identifying relevant ones can be a time-consuming process. Indeed, even if your newsreader client supports keyword searching of newsgroup titles, relevant groups may still be overlooked. A title search for a newsgroup on prostatic hypertrophy for example, would not identify the group *sci.med.prostate.bhp* (bhp is the acronym for benign prostatic hypertrophy).

In recognition of this problem, the Usenet Info Center has been established to allow users to search a database of newsgroup descriptions. A search for the phrase 'repetitive strain injury' for example, indicates that the *sci.med.occupation* newsgroup caters for this speciality. This search engine can be reached at:

http://sunsite.unc.edu/usenet-i/search.html

This resource also presents users with the option to read any FAQs (a list of frequently asked questions) that a newsgroup may have generated. FAQs are devised in an attempt to minimise the posting of questions that have been sent and answered many times before. The FAQ that accompanies the *sci.med.aids* newsgroup, for example, provides answers to questions such as 'How is AIDS transmitted?', 'Are alternative treatments available?' and 'Where can I find out more information about AIDS?'

Newsgroup netiquette dictates that relevant FAQs are read *before* questions are posted. Failure to comply with this recommendation may lead to some fairly inflammatory comments ending up in your mailbox.

A final approach to identifying a speciality-

Table 6.1 Newsgroup hierarchy

	Topic	Example
alt	Alternative	*alt.comics.batman*
bionet	Biology	*bionet.microbiology*
comp	Computers	*comp.sys.mac.graphics*
misc	Miscellaneous	*misc.jobs.offered*
news	Topics on Usenet newsgroups	*news.groups.questions*
rec	Recreational	*rec.collecting.stamps*
sci	Sciences	*sci.med.aids*
soc	Society – cultural	*soc.history.war.world-war-ii*
talk	Talk	*talk.politics.medicine*

relevant newsgroups is to search the newsgroup archives. However, because of the volume of newsgroup messages is estimated to be around one Gbyte a month, very few sites on the Internet offer this service.[12] One exception to this however, is DejaNews:

http://www.dejanews.com/

Searching this database for the acronym MRSA I discovered that the newsgroups *sci.med.nursing*, *sci.med.pharmacy* and *bionet.microbiology* had all had recent postings on this subject and thus were suitable for subscription (Figs 6.11, 6.12). The DejaNews database also provides hypertext links to specific items of news. As these are available from DejaNews, access to a 'news feed' server is not required.

Filtering the news

Though newsgroups can be interesting, informative and entertaining they are also very time-consuming. A typical newsgroup in the

sci.med hierarchy will generate around 20 postings a day. Though this number is manageable, if you subscribe to other equally active newsgroups and/or forget to collect the news on a particular day, it is not long before information overload is experienced.

In addition to this issue of quantity, there is also the problem of relevance. For example, if you are interested in following and participating in discussions on 'breast cancer' it would appear to make sense to subscribe to groups such as *sci.med.diseases.cancer* and *sci.med.pathology*. However, as both groups cover a fairly broad spectrum, it is probable that most of the discussion will *not* be focused on this speciality. If this scenario were not bad enough, there is the related problem that *other* newsgroups may carry postings on breast cancer that you would miss. A search on the DejaNews database indicates that the groups *sci.med*, *sci.environmnet*, *bionet.general* and *sci.psychology.misc* regularly carry postings on this topic.

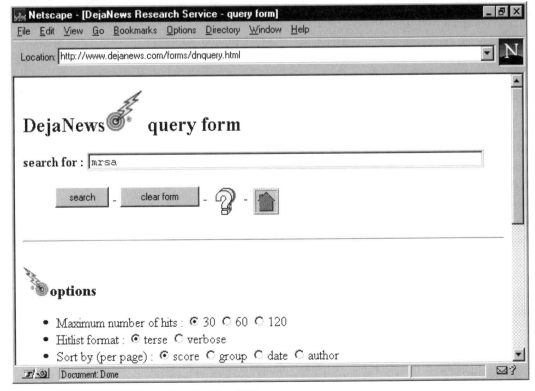

Fig. 6.11 A search of the DejaNews database for MRSA

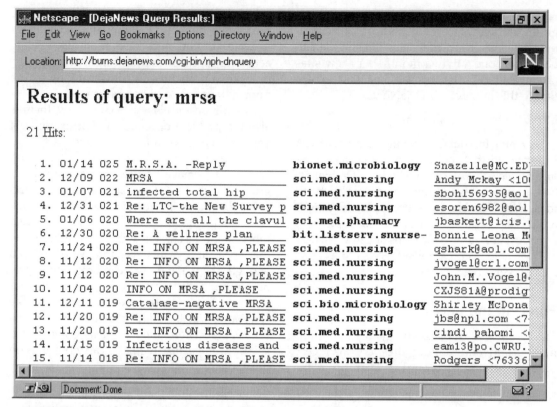

Fig. 6.12 Results of the search for MRSA: the newsgroup *sci.med.nursing* looks like a good source of information for this subject

One solution to these problems is to cancel your newsgroup subscriptions and replace them with a personal commitment to search the DejaNews database on a day-by-day basis.

A less labour-intensive and more practical solution though is to establish a newsgroup search profile with the EBInet Biosciences NetNews Filtering Service. This service automatically sifts *all* the newsgroup mailings posted within the biology or scientific hierarchy, looking for any articles that match your search profile. When a match is made, the original newsgroup message is automatically sent to your electronic mailbox.

To ensure that you only receive relevant articles, it is imperative that you define a good search profile. Typically, this will require you to define which words should and should not appear in the mailed articles. For example, the profile 'breast cancer not HRT' will find newsgroup messages where breast cancer is dis-cussed but HRT is not mentioned (Fig. 6.13). When a particularly relevant article has been found, you can use the relevance feedback utility to further improve your defined search profile.

To access the EBINet Biosciences NetNews Filtering Service point your Web browser at:

http://www.ebi.ac.uk/sift/

CONCLUSION

A recent article in the *BMJ* drew attention to the fact that patients were beginning to use e-mail to communicate with health professionals.[13] Leaving aside issues such as whether or not this medium is appropriate for sensitive and confidential data, this highlights the fact that e-mail has become an accepted and popular mode of communication.

In addition to facilitating the doctor/patient

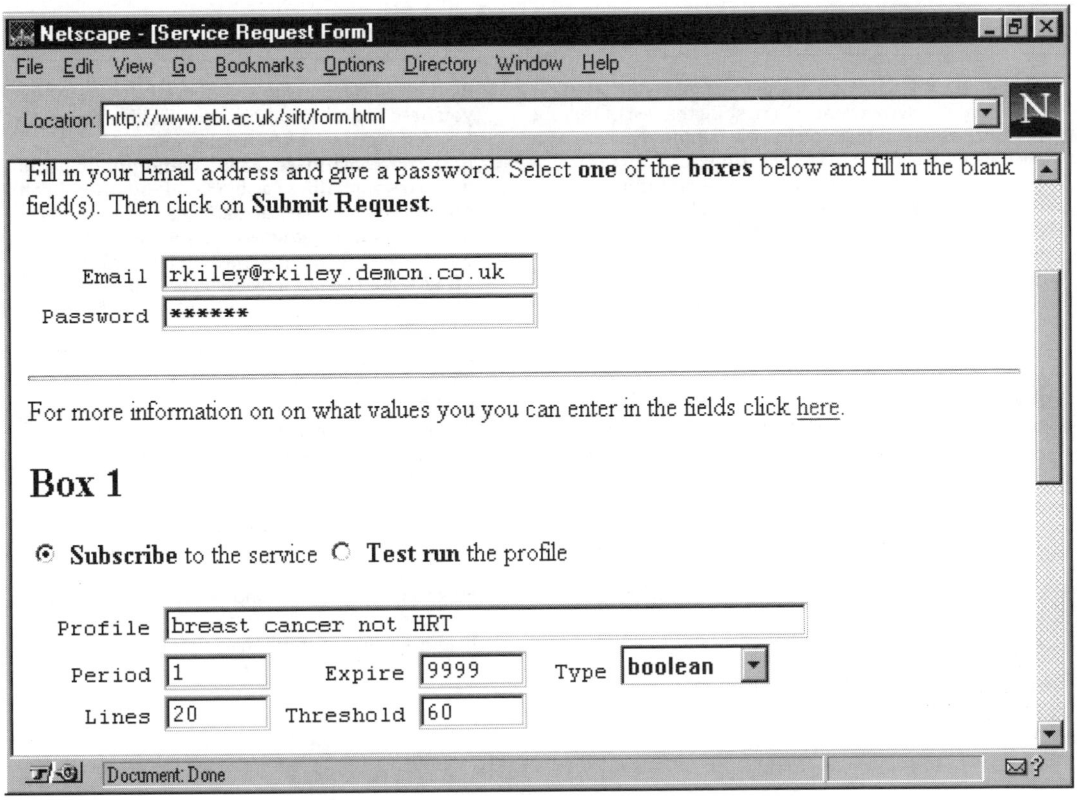

Fig. 6.13 Defining a newsgroup search profile with the EBINet BioSci Netnews Filtering Service

relationship, studies also show that doctor/doctor relationships are enhanced by e-mail. A study by Singarella et al found that doctors working in two health sciences institutions used e-mail in preference to the telephone or the traditional letter. With e-mail, response rates were deemed to be quicker and communication errors reduced.[14]

This chapter has demonstrated how e-mail is used to communicate on a group-wide basis through discussion lists and newsgroups. Despite the obvious benefits these can deliver to health professionals, it is important to remember that the quality of information posted in these forums is highly variable. In the light of this, I suspect that there will be an increasing tendency to establish physician-only discussion lists where the quality of the questions and answers can be assured. It should also be emphasised that, in this litigation-minded world, newsgroup or discussion list postings that request help in diagnosing or treating a particular medical condition should be ignored, or answered with disclaimers that would render future legal action futile.

Having drawn attention to these concerns, I would still urge all health professionals to participate in Internet-based group discussions. Providing you select your lists and newsgroups with care, you will find them informative, interesting and enjoyable.

REFERENCES AND NOTES

1 Though such services are of use to people who have a "mail-only" Internet connection, since the rest of this book has assumed that you have a full Internet connection, with a World Wide Web browser, I am not going to detail how these tasks can be performed by e-mail. If you require this information then obtain a copy of Bob Rankin's *Guide to Offline Internet Access* by sending the following message:

To:	mailbase@mailbase.ac.uk
Subject:	*leave blank*
Text:	send lis-iis e-access-inet.txt

If your mailer automatically appends a signature to your mail, disable this function for this message.

2 Anon. Threat to mail as macro viruses sweep the world. Personal Computer World December 1995 p. 18

3 Evidence-based health is a Mailbase discussion list. To subscribe send the following message:

To:	mailbase@mailbase.ac.uk
Subject:	*leave blank*
Text:	Subscribe evidence-based-health *firstname surname*

4 *gp-uk* is a Mailbase discussion list. To subscribe send the following message:

To:	mailbase@mailbase.ac.uk
Subject:	*leave blank*
Text:	Subscribe gp-uk *firstname surname*

5 Before you can join the VASCUNET discussion list you need to seek clearance from the list moderator Al Lossing. Address: alossing@hookup.net

6 http://www.mailbase.ac.uk/lists-p-t/public-health/

7 http://www.mailbase.ac.uk/lists-k-o/nukop-health/

8 http://www.mailbase.ac.uk/#lists

9 http://www.tile.net/news/newsnewu.html

10. http://www.tile.net/news/scimedai.html
http://www.tile.net/news/scimedte.html

11 A public news server is accessible from the following address:
gopher://gopher.bham.ac.uk/11/Usenet
Note Users outside Birmingham University cannot post messages to a group.

12 'DejaNews provide access to most of the Usenet Newsgroup postings which have appeared in the preceding four weeks – a single database of over 4 Gbytes of data':
http://www.dejanews.com/dnbig.html

13 Sellu D. Clinical encounters in cyberspace. British Medical Journal 1996 312:49

14 Singarella T, Baxter J, Sandefur R R, Emery C C. The effects of electronic mail on communication in two health sciences institutions. Journal of Medical Systems 1993 17 (2): 69–86

7

The future

Box 7.1 Chapter objectives

- Look at some of the new tools for health
  professionals that are emerging on the
  Internet.

- Examine whether the Internet infrastructure –
  the wires and cables – is big enough to satisfy
  current and future demand for Internet
  services.

- Discuss some of the ethical issues the Internet
  poses for health professionals.

INTRODUCTION

The cliché that 'the only certainty is change'
succinctly captures the essence of the Internet.
Beginning in 1969 as a network of just four
computers, the Internet has evolved into a
world wide network linking some 9 million
computers and around 30 million people.[1,2]

Impressive though these figures are, they
belie the fact that most of this growth has
taken place within the past 2 years following
the release of *Mosaic*, the first graphical World
Wide Web browser.[3] This development not
only altered the way the Internet looked, but
more fundamentally it changed peoples' per-
ceptions of what it could be used for. Virtually
overnight, the difficult, user-hostile command-line interface was replaced by one that
could play audio clips, display videos and
images, contain links to related documents,
and in a more recent development, run other
computer programs and applications. As it
has become easier to use, more people have
sought access. In turn, this has encouraged
even more companies and institutions to
make their resources available on the Internet.

In many ways, these developments have been mirrored in the arena of medical information. Though by 1993, resources such as those at the National Institutes of Health and the National Library of Medicine could be accessed through applications like <u>Gopher</u> and <u>Telnet</u>, the majority of sites that have been discussed in this book had no presence on the Internet. Moreover, the idea that you could use the Internet to simulate an interactive patient encounter, or attend a virtual conference were still considered to be the stuff of science fiction. Within the space of 2 years both of these ideas, and countless others, have been realised.

This chapter looks at new uses of the Internet in the context of health care, and indicates how these are being used to improve patient care. In discussing these, we also look at some of the technical and ethical issues that the Internet currently poses.

MEDICAL DECISION SUPPORT SYSTEMS

In an attempt to minimise the incidence of misdiagnosis, physicians are increasingly looking to decision support systems to corroborate their findings and/or highlight anomalies and errors. In recent months, some of these support systems have begun to appear on the Internet; three of the most significant are described below.

Cardiac Arrhythmia Advisory System

http://wailer.uokhsc.edu/einthoven.html

The specialist knowledge required to accurately interpret ECG results means that this work is usually performed in hospitals or dedicated cardiac units. Recognising that this situation is not always convenient for the patient – particularly in rural areas of the

United States where the nearest hospital may be several hours' drive – staff at the University of Oklahoma Health Sciences Center have developed the *Cardiac Arrhythmia Advisory System (CAAS). CAAS* is a computer program that can *expertly* analyse and interpret ECGs.

Using this Internet-based service, general practitioners can now record an ECG in their own surgery and FTP it to the CAAS server for analysis. The *CAAS* system then generates a series of outputs including a beat-by-beat analysis, a copy of the original tracing and an image of the ECG that can be interrogated. For example, by mouse-clicking wave 11 (Fig. 7.1) the system reports that 'this is ventricular activation. It arises from wave 10 during sinus rhythm'.

With the current trend in the UK and elsewhere to transfer patient services from the hospital to the community, and the finding which suggests that 75% of general practitioners are unable to correctly interpret non-acute abnormalities from an ECG, the development of computerised decision support tools such as this, is most timely.[4]

Hepaxpert

http://www.ping.at/hepax

The *Hepaxpert* program makes available precise and exhaustive interpretations of hepatitis serologic results. Via a World Wide Web form, the user inputs the results of a hepatitis test and submits this for analysis (Fig. 7.2). Results are returned by <u>e-mail</u> within 24 hours.

As the knowledge base of *Hepaxpert* contains 13 'if-then' rules for hepatitis A, and 106 rules for hepatitis B serology, all possible combinations of serologic test results – including rare and complex ones – can be interpreted. These rules also allow improbable and even impossible test results to be identified.

Thus, on submitting the hepatitis B serology results shown in Table 7.1, *Hepaxpert* reported that:

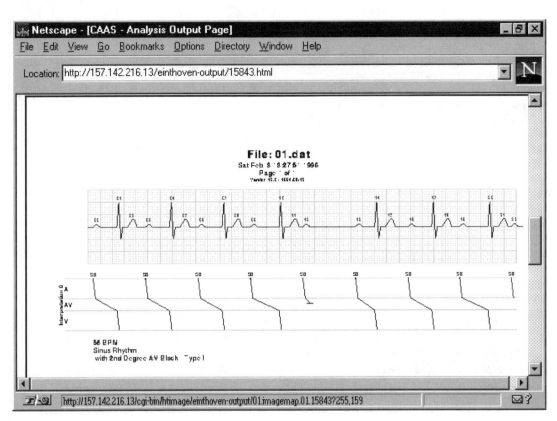

Fig. 7.1   *CAA*: analysis output page

the simultaneous occurrence of HBs-antigen and anti-HBs antibodies, with negative IgM anti-HBc antibodies, is a rare event in the natural course of a hepatitis B virus infection. This constellation of findings may be attributed to one of the following causes: (a) circulating HBsAg-anti-HBs immune complexes, (b) hepatitis B virus infection coinciding with a hepatitis B vaccination or injection of HB-hyperimmune globulin, or (c) reinfection with a hepatitis virus B with a different HBsAg subtype. Blood and secretions (saliva, sperm, breast milk) of such patients are to be regarded as infectious.

If the turn-around time for results is unacceptable, a copy of the *Hepaxpert* program can be purchased. The price and ordering details are available from the Web page cited above.

Table 7.1   Hepatitis B test results: sent to *Hepaxpert* for analysis

Test	Result
HBsAg	Positive
Anti-HBs	Positive
Anti-HBc	Negative
IgM anti-HBc	Negative
HBeAg	Borderline
Anti-HBe	Borderline

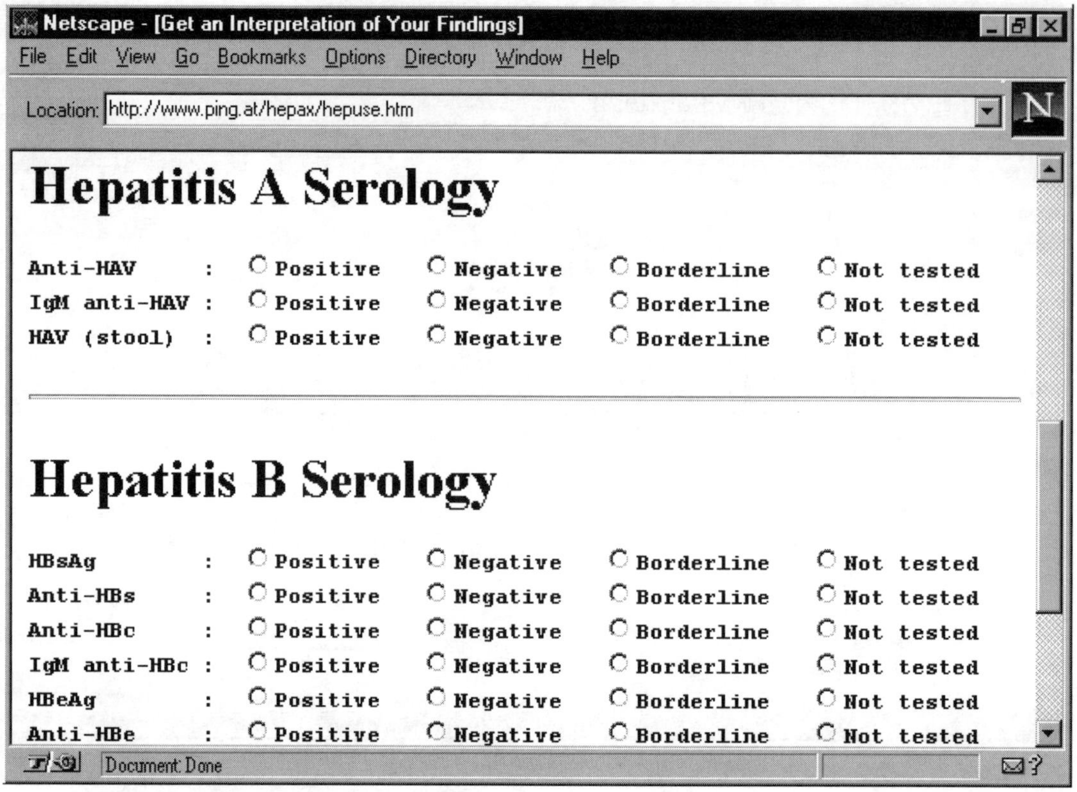

Netscape - [Get an Interpretation of Your Findings]

File   Edit   View   Go   Bookmarks   Options   Directory   Window   Help

Location: http://www.ping.at/hepax/hepuse.htm

Hepatitis A Serology

Anti-HAV   :   ○ Positive   ○ Negative   ○ Borderline   ○ Not tested
IgM anti-HAV :   ○ Positive   ○ Negative   ○ Borderline   ○ Not tested
HAV (stool)   :   ○ Positive   ○ Negative   ○ Borderline   ○ Not tested

Hepatitis B Serology

HBsAg   :   ○ Positive   ○ Negative   ○ Borderline   ○ Not tested
Anti-HBs   :   ○ Positive   ○ Negative   ○ Borderline   ○ Not tested
Anti-HBc   :   ○ Positive   ○ Negative   ○ Borderline   ○ Not tested
IgM anti-HBc :   ○ Positive   ○ Negative   ○ Borderline   ○ Not tested
HBeAg   :   ○ Positive   ○ Negative   ○ Borderline   ○ Not tested
Anti-HBe   :   ○ Positive   ○ Negative   ○ Borderline   ○ Not tested

Document: Done

Fig. 7.2   *Hepaxpert*. WWW analysis submission form

Columbia Clinical Information System

http://www.cpmc.columbia.edu/cisdemo

This Web-based product, developed by the Department of Medical Informatics at Columbia University, is an excellent example of how the Internet can be used in *conjunction* with a patient administration system (PAS) to create a fully integrated decision support system.

In common with most other computerised patient administration systems, the *Columbia Clinical Information System (CCIS)* records the patient's name, hospital number, date of birth and gender (Fig. 7.3). In addition to this, the clinician can also find what surgical and/or laboratory procedures have been performed, and access discharge summaries and radiological reports. As this data is all viewed via a Web browser, it is also possible for staff to view ECGs, X-rays, and CT scans.

Though this wealth of data obtainable through one application demonstrates the versatility of the Web browser, this is not the real strength of *CCIS*. What differentiates this system from others, is the way the clinician can link patient data to other sources of information to build up a better understanding of the clinical problem (Figs 7.4, 7.5). This concept is best illustrated by example in Box 7.2.

Though the *CCIS* does not go beyond the point reached in Box 7.2, it would not be difficult to set up links to full-text journal databases or to document delivery systems.

Thus, using just *one* interface from *one* computer workstation a complete patient record can be accessed, and when further information is needed to enhance this data, external databases held on the Internet can be automatically searched. The 'one-stop' clinical information system has clearly arrived.

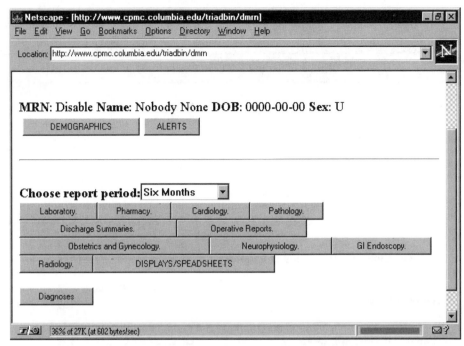

Fig. 7.3 *CCIS*: the entire patient record is accessible through this Web interface

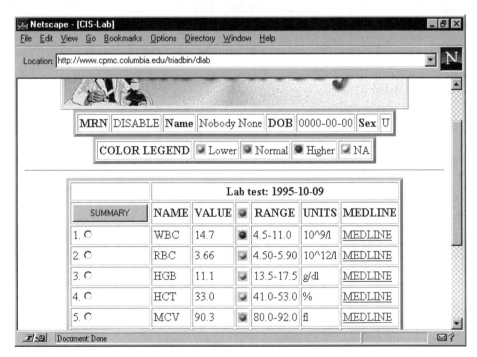

Fig. 7.4 *CCIS* displays the laboratory results of the ABC tests: WBC – white blood cell count – is high

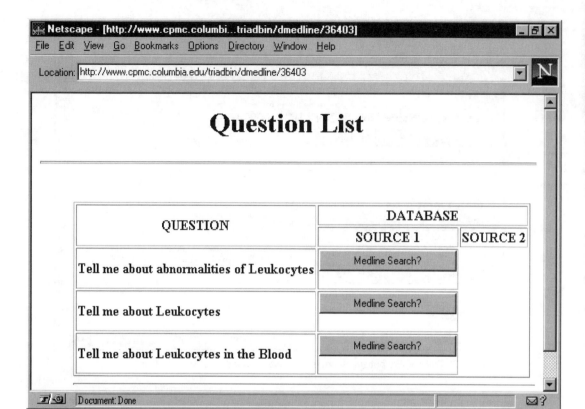

Fig. 7.5 *CCIS* generates a series of questions for the MEDLINE database to help the clinician find more information about the implications of the high WBC count

---

Box 7.2 Working with *CCIS*

A doctor accesses a patient's record to see what laboratory tests have been performed and what their results were.

Methodology
As this information is displayed, the expert computer system also alerts the doctor to other related information sources. (This is achieved by consulting the Medical Entities Dictionary – a clinical thesaurus.) If, for example, the doctor had been looking at a serum sodium test, the expert system would indicate that 'sodium' is related to 'hypernatremia'.

By determining related concepts, the program is able to generate questions to applications on the Internet such as MEDLINE, Physicians Desk Reference, and DXplain. In this example, the expert system offered the doctor the option to run a search on MEDLINE to find out about abnormalities of sodium in the serum or to ask DXplain about the symptoms of hypernatremia. In both cases, all the doctor has to do is select which search to execute. The doctor does *not* have to devise the search strategy. Within a short time, the results of the search are displayed through the Web browser.

Note For reasons of patient confidentiality the demonstration version of this expert system contains just one patient record from which all personal details have been removed.

TELEMEDICINE

Telemedicine can be defined as the use of telecommunications technologies to facilitate healthcare delivery. Dating back to the 1920s, when ship-to-shore radios were used by doctors to assist with medical emergencies at sea, telemedicine has advanced to the point where remote doctor–doctor or doctor–patient consultations can now occur over the Internet.

One of the most exciting examples of this is the *TeleMed* system, developed for the National Jewish Center for Immunology and Respiratory Medicine (NJC) in Denver, Colorado.

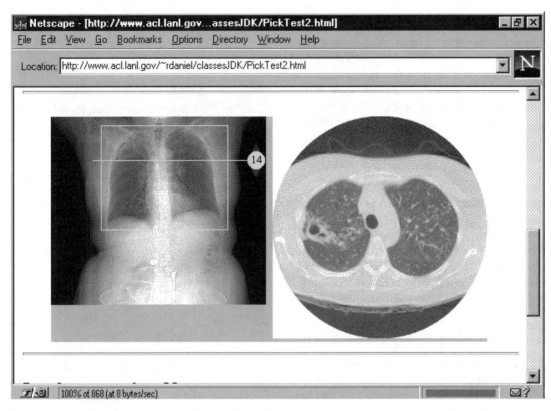

Fig. 7.6 A Java applet: when any part of the frontal X-ray is selected, the corresponding slice is displayed in the adjacent panel

TeleMed

**http://www.acl.lanl.gov/~rdaniel/
classesJDK/PickTest2.html**

The purpose of project *TeleMed*, which has been given the appellation 'the virtual patient record system' is to make the knowledge and experience of the pulmonary specialists at the NJC available to a wider audience. To achieve this, staff at 'non-specialist centres' FTP chest X-rays to a national radiographic repository. Specialists from the NJC then retrieve these images and analyse them.

What makes this telemedicine system unique is the fact that the retrieved X-rays are delivered to the Web browser as a Java applet. (A Java applet is a computer program that can be included on an HTML page.) In this case, the Java applet displays two images; a frontal X-ray and a transverse slice from part of the lung. When any part of the frontal X-ray is selected by pointing and clicking with your mouse, the corresponding slice is displayed in the adjacent panel (Fig. 7.6).

Highly trained specialists are an expensive and scarce resource. Telemedical applications such as this help to ensure that these resources are used effectively.

THE INFORMATION SUPERHIGHWAY

The increasing reliance on the Internet for mail, information, education, and decision-support, raises the issue of whether or not the network infrastructure is sufficiently developed to handle this volume of traffic. To assess this, we can examine current developments in both public and institutional computer networks.

Public networks

Unless you are part of an institution that has a dedicated 'feed' to the Internet (discussed below) the only way you can access the Internet is by setting up an account with a commercial Internet provider. Once this has been established, you can access their Internet 'feed' via the telephone network (Ch. 2).

Though this mode of access is perfectly acceptable, indeed most of the research for this book was undertaken using a <u>dial-up</u> connection, as the Internet moves increasingly away from text-based sources to high-bandwidth multimedia applications, the relative slowness of the telephone connection will be exacerbated. Thus, whereas most commercial Internet providers are connected to the Internet at speeds of between 64 <u>kbps</u> (kilobits per second) and 2 <u>Mbps</u> (megabits per second), their customers (you and I) are connected by a modem running at either 14.4 kbps or 28.8 kbps. Like any system, the Internet is as only as good as its weakest link; at the moment this is represented by the telephone line.

The obvious solution to this problem of access speed is the creation of a national high-speed computer network. In the United States, such a plan is being enabled through the National Information Infrastructure (NII).

National Information Infrastructure

The NII aims to connect every home, business and school in the United States to the high-speed network thereby 'unleashing an information revolution that will change forever the way people live, work and interact with each other'. Paramount to this project is the explicit objective that information resources will be 'available to all at affordable prices'. In more visionary tones, the NII *Agenda for Action* concludes, 'Because information means empowerment – and employment-the government has a duty to ensure that all Americans have access to the resources and job creation potential of the Information Age'.[5]

In stark contrast, the UK government has no plans to build a national high-speed computer network. As this situation is unlikely to change in the immediate future, users who want faster access to the Internet must look elsewhere.

ISDN and broadband technology

One way UK Internet users can increase access speed is to use the Integrated Service Digital Network (ISDN). This network supports speeds of 128 kbps – 4 to 5 times quicker than the fastest modem. Moreover as this network is digital – in contrast to the telephone network which is analogue – data transfer is more reliable.

The only problem with ISDN is cost. British Telecom, the providers of ISDN in the UK, charge £400.00 for installing an ISDN line and £84.00 per quarter for line rental. Call charges are the same as for a normal telephone line.[6] In addition to these costs, you need extra hardware to enable your computer to communicate over ISDN (around £300.00 for an ISDN terminal adaptor) *and* you pay an increased fee to your Internet provider. U-Net for example, an Internet provider that offers ISDN access, levies a one-off joining fee of £80.00 and a monthly subscription of £40.00. This compares with their standard modem access charges of £12.00 and £10.00 respectively.[7]

Though ISDN dramatically decreases data transfer time, it has been calculated that it would still take 24 hours to transfer a 60-minute video film.[8] Consequently, if users are to take full advantage of the emerging Internet services – high-quality video teaching for example – then broadband technology greater than that offered by ISDN is now required.

In the UK this is most likely to come via the cable television companies who are currently laying high-capacity coaxial cable to around 10 million homes. In conjunction with this, work is taking place to develop cable modems that will be able to deliver data at the rate of 10 Mbps. Though at the moment (February 1996) no cable company in the UK can offer this service, it seems likely that by the end of this year, or in early 1997 Internet access via this high speed cable network will be a possibility. For those homes that have access to this network, the information super-highway will become a reality.[9]

Institutional networks

NHS-wide network

For health professionals working in the UK, the most significant networking development is the creation of the NHS-wide network. Though its main purpose is administrative – to facilitate the growing need for organisations within the NHS to share information – details released so far indicate that the network will also provide a high-speed access point to the Internet. In addition to this, the network will host products that contribute to the knowledge base of health care. No definitive list has yet been published but it seems reasonable to assume that the Cochrane Database of Systematic Reviews and the databases produced by the NHS Centre for Reviews and Dissemination will be available via this network.

As the data on the NHS-wide network is highly sensitive and confidential, the network will not form part of the Internet. Internet access will be via a secure one-way gateway that will prevent ingress on to the NHS-wide network from Internet users.

The NHS-wide network is still very much in its developmental stage; indeed it has not gone 'live' at the time of writing. For the latest information on this project, contact the NHS-wide network help line on:

44 (0)121 625 3838

SuperJANET

For academics in the UK, the problem of access speed is being addressed with the development of SuperJANET, an advanced high-speed optical computer network. When fully implemented, data will be distributed across this network at speeds of around 600 Mbps; a 300-fold increase in performance when compared with the existing JANET network.[10]

One example of how this high-speed net-work is being used in the field of medical education is the Interactive Teaching Project in Surgery, developed by University College, London.[11] Via this initiative, medical students at five SuperJANET sites can watch live transmissions of surgical operations and interact with the surgical team as if they were actually in the operating theatre. Thus, this project allows a large number of students to see a wide range of operative procedures and hear and see at first hand the opinions and skills of some of the best surgeons in the UK.

National Research and Education Network

In the United States high-speed networking for the academic and research community is being facilitated through the National Research and Education Network (NREN). Even faster than SuperJANET, NREN will eventually be able to deliver access speeds of 2.5 Gbps (gigabits per second). [12]

Whichever way you access the Internet, it is a fairly safe assumption that over the next few years *all* routes will get faster and more reliable. It is, however, an equally safe assumption that in parallel with this, bigger and more sophisticated applications will also be developed. Whether or not the network infrastructure will keep pace with these, remains to be seen.

THE INTERNET AND THE PATIENT: ETHICAL DILEMMAS

In the main, providing health information has been the exclusive prerogative of health professionals. Individuals who try to find information about a specific illnesses or disease are often restricted to joining a self-help group or asking friends and colleagues. The hospital library – the obvious reference place – is usually reserved for health professionals, and though public libraries may be more welcoming, their collection of medical literature may not be particularly good. Despite the universal interest in health, few public libraries take even the most popular medical journals, such as the *BMJ*, or the *New England*

Journal of Medicine, and fewer still offer their users access to databases like MEDLINE.

Though recent initiatives in the UK, such as the Health Information Service, have highlighted the need to make health information more accessible, evidence tends to suggest that these needs are still un-met.[13]

The Internet has the potential to reverse this situation. A great wealth of medical information is as freely available to the general public as it is to health professionals. Moreover, with the development of freenets – organisations who provide free Internet access to the public – this information becomes available to all, irrespective of socio-economic status. In the UK, the Croydon Public Library Service is the first authority to establish a free Internet service.[14]

Widespread access to health information, however, will exacerbate existing conflicts between patients' expectations of health care and what the system can afford to deliver. For example, a multiple sclerosis patient who searches the Internet for information about this condition will, with very little effort, find the following:

The Food and Drug Administration (FDA) recently approved Betaseron (human interferon-beta) for use in selected patients with multiple sclerosis (MS) basing their decision on a well designed clinical trial. In that trial the drug was demonstrated to reduce the relapse rate of certain remitting-relapsing patients and to decrease MRI evidence of MS activity in the brain.[15]

As this research was published by the American Academy of Neurology (AAN) the source can be considered authoritative.

Betaseron, however, does not come cheap. The cost of one year's treatment is around £10 000. Taking the AAN figures that this drug would help about 45% of those with the disease, the total cost of treating this proportion of UK multiple sclerosis patients would be £380 million a year – about 10% of the total national drugs bill.[16] Despite claims by successive Secretaries of State for Health that patients will always receive the drugs they need, it is difficult to believe that available resources would permit this level of expenditure. Consequently, the rationing of health

care that has *always* existed will, as a consequence of the Internet, become more transparent.

It can also be anticipated that as patients become more aware of new, alternative, and better treatment options, more doctors will find themselves subjected to charges of medical negligence. In law, negligence is defined as 'the breach of duty to use reasonable care, as a result of which there is damage to another'.[17] To prove this, it must be shown that, on the balance of all probabilities, injury to the patient resulted from the negligent act of the doctor.

In the context discussed here, a doctor could be sued for negligence if the treatment given to a patient was contrary to accepted best practice. Referring back to the example in Box 3.2, a doctor could be sued for negligence if he continued to prescribe high doses of nifedipine (80 mg or greater) to treat hypertension, angina, or myocardial infarction when there is clear and *accessible* evidence that this treatment significantly increases mortality.[18]

Also, as more individuals get Internet access and subscribe to the various health-related newsgroups and discussion lists, it is likely that doctors will have to spend more time counselling patients who have read some misleading or erroneous item. Informing patients of *authoritative* sources of health information may be one of the new responsibilities the Internet will impose on health professionals.

CONCLUSION

The future of the Internet is one where change and evolution are its constant bedfellows. The widespread introduction of voice-mail for example, looks likely to be the next big application to take hold on the Internet, whilst in more general terms, users can expect services to become increasingly commercialised.

For health professionals, the Internet of the future will offer enhanced access to a wealth of information resources and teaching tools, and, through telemedical applications and decision support systems, will provide the opportunity to deliver patient care more effectively.

The size and volatility of the Internet ensures that any book on this subject can only provide a snapshot of what is available. To explore further, and truly reap the benefits that the Internet can deliver, I urge all health professionals to get connected, and get connected now!

Finally, I would like to remind you that many of the key Internet sites discussed in this text can be accessed from the Churchill Livingstone World Wide Web site at:

http://www.churchillmed.com/BOOKS/ medinter.html

From this page you can also mail me with comments and questions, and suggest other interesting Internet sites that could be included in future editions.

I look forward to hearing from you.

REFERENCES AND NOTES

1 http://www.nw.com/
2 http://www1.mids.org/growth/internet/hosts.dog
gopher://akasha.tic.com:70/00/matrix/news/v5/press
957.509
3 The Internet Domain Survey, conducted by NetWizards in January 1996, shows that in January 1994 the number of host computers on the Internet was just over 2 million. In January 1996, this figure soared to 9.4 million:
http://www.nw.com/zone/WWW/report.html
4 McCrea W A, Saltissi S Electrocardiogram interpretation in general practice: relevance to prehospital thrombolysis. British Heart Journal 1993 70 (3):219–225
5 http://sunsite.unc.edu/nii/NII-Executive-Summary.html
6 Prices correct, February 1996
7 www.u-net.com/services/e3ip.htm
8 Winder D Step up to the superhighway. Sunday Times (newspaper) 7 January 1996 at:
http://www.sunday-times.co.uk/
9 Though some cable companies are already offering Internet access, this is via the telephone network, rather than the high-speed cable network. A spokesman from CableTel (a cable franchisee in the UK) indicated that 'the race was on' to see which company could offer Internet access via this high-speed network.
10 http://www.ukerna.ac.uk/SuperJANET/SuperJANET/SuperJANET-Intro/Introduction.html
11 http://av.avc.ucl.ac.uk/tltp/insurrect.html
12 http://www.hpcc.gov/blue94/section.3.2.html
13 Buckland S Unmet needs for health information: a literature review. Health Libraries Review 1994 11 (2):82–95
14 http://clip.croydon.gov.uk/contents.html
15 http://synapse.uah.ualberta.ca/aan/000p0000.htm
16 Walley T, Barton S A purchaser perspective of managing new drugs: interferon beta as a case study. British Medical Journal 1995 311 (7008):796–799
17 British Medical Association Rights and responsibilities of doctors. BMJ Publishing 1992 p. 19
18 http://www.medtext.com/newsal.htm

Finding more information

If after reading this book you would like to learn more about the Internet, the sources below are recommended starting points. For ease of use I have split these resources into two sections. First, those resources that can be accessed via the Internet. Secondly, for readers who have not yet got connected, I have compiled a brief, annotated bibliography.

INTERNET RESOURCES

Tutorials

These two resources are Internet-based courses that aim to help new users make effective use of the Internet. Both are free of charge and may be undertaken at your own pace.

The Online Netskills Interactive Course (TONIC)

http://www.netskills.ac.uk/TONIC/

TONIC is a Web-based interactive tutorial designed to offer practical guidance on how to use the Internet. The main modules of the course are:

- exploring the Internet;
- basic network operations – Telnet, and FTP;
- searching the Internet;
- communicating via the Internet.

Which of these you pursue, or in what order is entirely up to you. Once you have registered your interest to follow this tutorial, you are assigned a log-in name. When you next log on, the program will remember which parts of the tutorial you have already completed.

This tutorial was produced as part of the ITTI Network Training Materials Project (NTMP) with some additional funding and support from other sources. Copyright of the course resides with Netskills, at the University of Newcastle.

Patrick Crispen's Internet Roadmap

http://www.brandonu.ca/~ennsnr/Resources/Roadmap/Welcome.html

Roadmap is another Internet training workshop designed to teach new 'net travellers' how to navigate the 'information superhighway'. Originally designed as a 6-week course conducted by e-mail, *Roadmap* has now been converted into hypertext and stored on the Web for easy access.

Discussion lists

Internet Tourbus

For suggestions on interesting Internet sites to visit, subscribe to the Internet Tourbus discussion list. Recommended sites come with an in-depth description and analysis. In an average month, the owners of the list will mail you with about five suggestions.

To subscribe, send the e-mail shown in Figure A.1.

NewbieNewz

This discussion list exists to serve the needs of new Internet users. Regular mailings aim to answer most questions new users are likely to ask; on those occasions when *specific* help is required, subscribers can mail the help desk for assistance.

To:	listserv@listserv.aol.com
Subject:	*leave blank*
Text:	subscribe tourbus *firstname surname*

Fig. A.1   How to subscribe to Internet Tourbus

To:	Majordomo@Newbie.NET
Subject:	*leave blank*
Text:	subscribe newbienewz *firstname surname*

Fig. A.2   How to subscribe to NewbieNewz

To subscribe to this mailing list send the e-mail shown in Figure A.2.

NON-INTERNET RESOURCES
Books

The number of books that discuss the Internet is staggering. A search of the Whitaker's *Books in Print* database identifies over 500 books on this topic, 60% of which have been published within the past year. I am, however, going to recommend just two:

- Schofield S *The UK Internet book revised for '95*. Addison-Wesley, 1995, ISBN 0201877317
- Krol E *The whole Internet: users guide and catalogue*, 2nd edn. O'Reilly & Associates, 1994, ISBN 1565920635

The first is aimed at the dial-up UK Internet market and provides an excellent introduction to the Internet.

The second is known as the 'Internet bible' and is still the most authoritative text available. It is, however, somewhat dated. Most of the examples assume you will be accessing the Internet through a command-line interface rather than a graphical one such as a Web browser.

Journals

To keep abreast of Internet developments, I would recommend subscribing to at least one Internet journal. The titles below are the ones that I find most useful. The general interest magazine *.net* is aimed at the UK Internet market, whilst *Medicine on the Net* concentrates on medical resources and applications on the Internet.

.net
Future Publishing Ltd, 30 Monmouth Street, Bath BA1 2BW
Tel: 44(0)1225 442244; Fax: 44(0)1225 423212
http://www.futurenet.co.uk/net.html
e-mail: netmag@futurenet.co.uk
ISSN: 1355–7602

Medicine on the Net
COR Healthcare Resources, PO Box 40959, Santa Barbara, CA 93140–0959
Tel: +1 905 564 2177; Fax: +1 805 564–2146
http://www.mednet-i.com
e-mail: mednet@corhealth.com
ISSN 1085–3502

Articles

A search of the MEDLINE database for the term 'Internet' indicates that in 1995, this one database indexed more than 100 articles on this subject. Key citations from this search are detailed below.

Ellenberger B 1995 Navigating physician resources on the Internet. Canadian Medical Association Journal 152 (8):1303–1307

Glowniak J V 1995 Medical resources on the Internet. Annals of Internal Medicine 13:123–131

McEnery K W 1995 The Internet, World Wide Web and Mosaic. American Journal of Roentgenology 164 (2):469–473

Millman A, Lee N, Kealy K 1995 ABC of medical computing: the Internet. British Medical Journal 311:440–443

Pallen M, Guide to the Internet. A series of four articles:

   (i)   Introducing the Internet. British Medical Journal 1995, 311:1422–1424

   (ii)   Electronic mail. British Medical Journal 1995, 311: 1487–1490

   (iii)   The world wide web. British Medical Journal 1995, 311: 1552–1556

   (iv)   Logging in, fetching files, reading news. British Medical Journal 1995, 311:1626–1630

Using Netscape Navigator

This appendix poses and answers the most frequently asked questions about installing, configuring and using _Netscape_ Navigator, the most popular World Wide Web browser. All commands are correct for _Netscape_ version 2.0, running under Window 3.x or Windows95.

Note In this appendix, commands appear in the form **Menuname | Command name**. Thus, **File | Save** means 'open the file menu and then select the save option'.

Where can I get the latest release of Netscape from?

To take advantage of the latest technological developments on the Internet, an up-to-date Web client is essential. For example, Java applets (computer programs that can be included on a Web page in much the same way as a graphic) can only be displayed if you are running version 2.0 (or later) of _Netscape_.

The latest version of _Netscape_ can always be obtained from:

http://home.netscape.com/

From this page, follow the links to the latest release appropriate to your operating system. (Windows95, Windows 3.1, Mac.) If a local mirror site is suggested use this for faster access.

Note A quick way to get to the Netscape Home Page is to click on the _Netscape_ icon displayed on every Web page. i.e. 'the flashing N'.

How long does it take to FTP Netscape?

As the size of the program varies between operating systems, I cannot give a definitive answer. As a guide, the version for Windows95 (3.192 MB in size) took around 35 minutes to FTP.

How do I install Netscape?

Netscape is delivered as a self-executable archive, and will be called something like 'n32e20.exe', depending on the version. Run this file to extract various files including a 'setup' file and a 'readme' file. Read the readme file, and then proceed with the set-up.

I get the message 'Cannot find Winsock' when I try to run Netscape. What does this mean?

As stressed in Chapter 2, when connecting to the Internet via a PC, you need to be running TCP/IP software. If you load *Netscape* before loading TCP/IP, you will receive the above message. To solve this, load TCP/IP before loading *Netscape*.

Netscape automatically loads the Netscape Home Page when I connect to the Internet. How I can stop this?

As shipped, *Netscape* is configured to load the *Netscape* Home Page. To stop this select **Options | General Preferences | Appearance | Start with blank page**.

To make the Churchill Livingstone Medical Information site your default home page select **Options | General Preferences | Appearance | Home Page Location** and enter

http://www.churchillmed.com/BOOKS/ medinter.html

How do I link to other pages and go back to a page I have already seen?

All highlighted words (coloured or underlined) are hypertext links. Clicking on any link will load up the related page, wherever it happens to be located on the Internet. Click on the arrow buttons ← → to go back or forward to another page. If your toolbar is not visible, select **Go | Forward** or **Go | Back**.

What are 'Bookmarks'?

Bookmarks are a way of recording the location of a particular Internet site. When you wish to revisit a book-marked site, you can do so without having to remember the specific URL.

How do I make a Bookmark?

To bookmark any page select **Bookmarks | Add Bookmark**. To arrange the Bookmarks hierarchically select **Bookmarks | Go to Bookmark | Insert Folder**. You can then cut and paste specific bookmark entries to specific folders. For example, you may have a 'Health' folder to keep health-related sites together and a search engine folder to facilitate easy access to your favourite search tools.

How can I save a file?

To minimise connect time, it makes sense to save files to disk. If you are viewing the file, click on **File | Save As** and assign a filename and location (or accept the default). To read this file when you have severed your connection to your Internet provider, select **File | Open File** and select the appropriate filename. To save a file to disk without viewing it first, click on any hypertext link with the Shift key held down.

How can I save an image?

When you save a file, images are replaced by icons. However, specific images can be saved by placing your mouse pointer over the image and clicking the right-hand mouse button. From the pop-up menu select '**Save this image as**' and enter a filename or accept the default.

How do I FTP a file with Netscape?

FTPing is the same process as saving a file (**File | Save As**). If you try to view a executable file (such as a program file) *Netscape* realises that the file cannot be displayed, and prompts you with a dialogue box to supply a filename and location.

How can I print a file?

If the *Netscape* tool bar is visible, press the printer icon; otherwise select **File | Print**. If this option is selected whilst you are connected to the Internet, images will be printed. As printing can be a relatively slow process (and therefore relatively costly) I would recommend saving the file to disk and printing it later.

When I try to connect to a Telnet site I get the message 'unable to find application'. What does this mean?

To run a Telnet session you must have a Telnet client, and configure *Netscape* to load this application. To do this select **Options | General Preferences | Apps | Supporting Applications | Telnet**. Give the filename and disk location of the Telnet client.

When I try to play a video through Netscape I get an 'application unknown' error message. What does this mean and how do I correct this?

Netscape can only display videos if you have a video client already installed on your computer. If this is the case you can configure *Netscape* to launch this application automatically. (This saves you the bother of having to save the file, and then load up another piece of software.) Select **Options | General Preferences | Helpers**. From the displayed list select the appropriate file type. In this example, select **video/mpeg**. In the bottom half of the window select the option **Launch the Application**. In the blank dialogue box enter the path and filename of your MPEG player. e.g. **c:\mpeg\mpeg.exe**

Whenever *Netscape* subsequently encounters an MPEG file it will automatically load the MPEG client. Chapter 3 has details on how to find software clients.

If I know the URL of a Web site can I jump straight to it?

Yes. Select **File | Open** and in the dialogue box type in the URL. Since most servers on the Internet are UNIX-based the case of the address is crucial. If an address is cited in lower case, and you enter it in capitals you will receive an error message to the effect that the address does not exist.

Note   As *Netscape* assumes that you are going to load an HTML file that uses the HTTP protocol (hypertext transfer protocol) the **http://** part of a Web address can be omitted. Thus **File | Open www.mailbase.ac.uk/** is the same as **File | Open http://www.mailbase.ac.uk/**

How can I speed up the loading of Web pages?

1   Disabling the image capabilities dramatically reduces the time it takes to load a Web page. This can be implemented by selecting **Options** and deselecting the **Auto Load Images** option. (This is a toggle switch; if the option is marked with a ✓ images will be displayed.) On those occasions when you want to see a specific image, simply click on the image's icon.

2. Some Internet providers set up a temporary cache to store all Web pages and files that have recently been accessed. If the Web site you want is already in this cache, then delivery to your desktop will be far quicker than if you have to fetch the page from the host server. To enable this service select **Options | Network Preferences | Proxies | Manual Proxy Configuration | View** and in the HTTP proxy box enter the address of this server, and its appropriate port. (This information will be supplied by your Internet provider.)

Despite using the cache, a particular Web page still seems to be taking a long time to come through. Can I stop the transfer?

Yes. Click the red 'Stop' button, if your *Netscape* toolbar is visible. Alternatively, select the **Go | Stop Loading** option or simply press the escape key on your keyboard.

Some of the graphics appear to be corrupted. Can I correct this?

Yes, by reloading the document through **View | Reload**.

How can I configure Netscape to send and receive e-mail?

To be able to send and receive mail through *Netscape* your Internet provider must provide *both* a SMTP (simple mail transfer protocol) server for outgoing mail and a POP3 (Post Office Protocol version 3) for incoming mail. If this is the case, then select **Options | Mail and News Preferences** and enter the address of the SMTP server, the POP3 server, and your POP3 user name in the appropriate boxes. Save these options.

To load the *Netscape Mail* client select **Window | Netscape Mail**. To retrieve mail from your provider's POP3 server select **File | Get New Mail**. To send messages select **File | Send Mail in Outbox**.

If your provider offers an SMTP server for both incoming and outgoing mail, *Netscape* can only be used to *send* mail. This is done through the **File | New Mail Message** option (Fig. B.1).

How can I configure Netscape to subscribe to and read Usenet Newsgroups?

To be able to subscribe to and read Usenet newsgroups your Internet provider must provide access to a NNTP (network news transport protocol) server. If this condition is met, select **Options | Mail and News Preferences** and enter the address of the NNTP server. The first time you connect to the NNTP server, *Netscape* will download a list of all available newsgroups.

To load the *Netscape News* browser select **Window | Netscape News**. To see which newsgroups are available for subscription select **Options | Show all Newsgroups**.

Can I search a Web page for a particular word or phrase?

Yes. Click on the binoculars option on your toolbar (or **Edit | Find**) and enter the word or phrase you wish to search for.

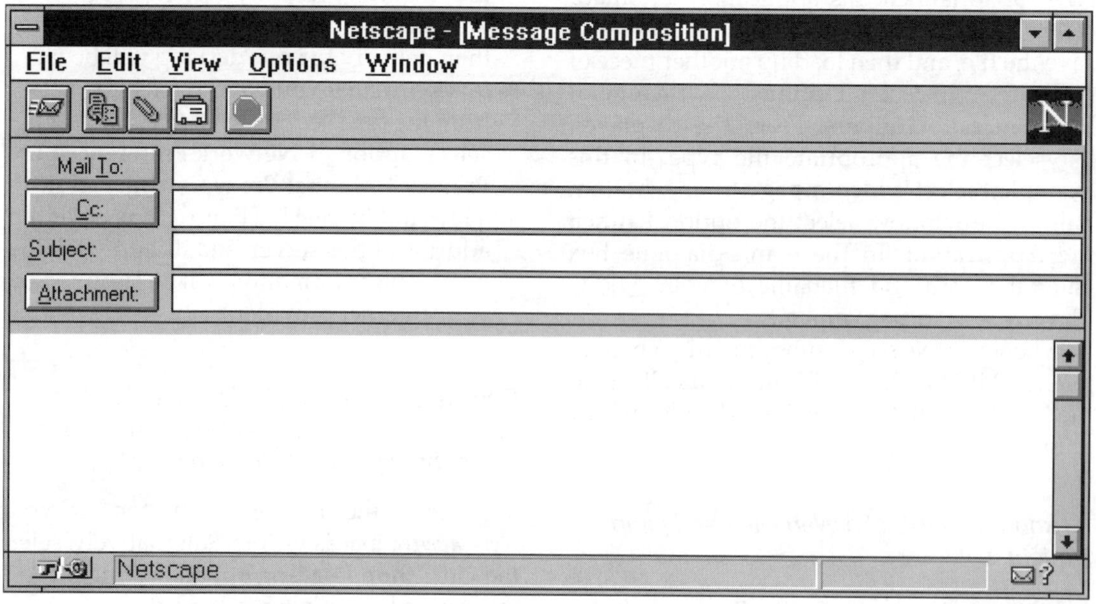

Fig. B.1 The *Netscape* e-mail client

What is the Network cache, and how do I empty it?

Pages received by *Netscape* are automatically cached to your computer's hard disk. Thus, when you want to go back to a page previously accessed (by pressing the ← arrow on the toolbar), *Netscape* can bring it back from the cache, rather than having to get it from the original server.

As this cache can get quite large, it is a good idea to empty it occasionally. To do this select **Options | Network Preferences | Clear disk cache now**. From this screen you will see that you have the opportunity to increase (or decrease) the size of the cache.

I want to purchase a product via the Internet; is it safe to transmit my credit card details through Netscape?

Yes, providing the site you are accessing uses the RSA public key cryptographic technology. This can be determined in three ways. First, the address will commence **https://** where the extra 's' means 'secure'. Secondly, in the bottom lefthand corner of every Web page viewed through *Netscape* there is a two-part key (Fig. B.2). If you connect to a secure site, the two halves of the key are joined up (Fig. B.3). Thirdly by selecting **View | Document Info** details of the security are shown (Fig. B.4).

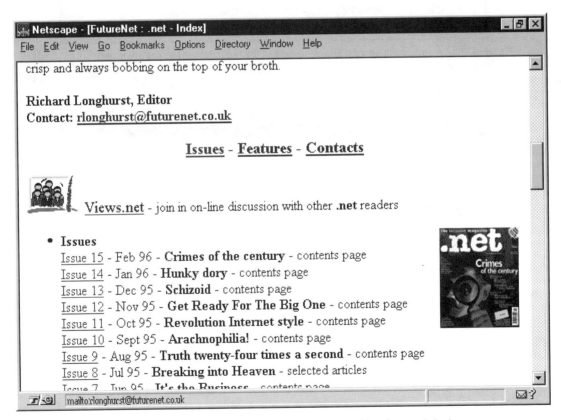

Fig. B.2 An insecure site as identified by *Netscape*: the key in the bottom lefthand corner is broken

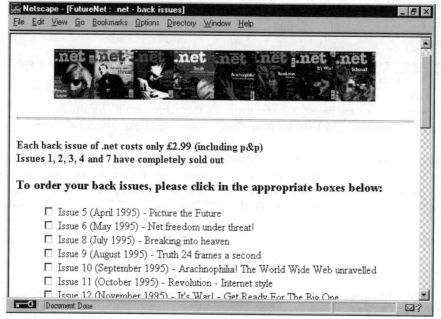

Fig. B.3   A secure site as identified by *Netscape*: the two halves of the key are joined

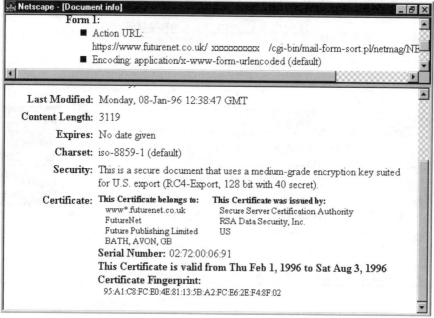

Fig. B 4   Document information details

Appendix C

Optimising your computer

This appendix describes a couple of 'tweaks' you can undertake to optimise your computer's performance for Internet-specific tasks.

UPGRADING THE PROCESSOR SERIAL PORT

The serial port is where you connect the modem to the computer. Generally speaking, to drive modems at speeds greater than 14 400 bps (bits per second), it is recommended that your serial port is fitted with a 16550A chip. How you check this depends on what sort of computer you have.

IBM-compatibles

For IBM compatibles, you need to get to the operating system (DOS) below Windows. To do this, follow these instructions.

1 Exit to DOS by closing Windows.
2 At the C: prompt type 'msd'. This will run the 'Microsoft Diagnostic Program'. If this file is not in your root directory, re-load Windows and use the search option within File Manager to identify the location of the file 'msd.exe'.
3 From the main diagnostic utility menu, select the option to examine the COM ports.
4 At the bottom of the display you will find notification of the type of UART chip each port uses. If an 8250 chip is reported, I would recommend upgrading. The cost of replacing this chip – around £25.00 – will be recovered through faster and, therefore, cheaper Internet sessions.

Other computers

For details of how to check the port settings on computers using other operating systems, either consult your manual or, once you have connected to the Internet, visit one of the following sites for further information:

Amiga Home Page
http://www.omnipresence.com/Amiga/ mainpage.html
Apple Home Page
http://www.info.apple.com
Atari Home Page
http://www.mcc.ac.uk/~dlms/atari.html

REVERSING DISK COMPRESSION UTILITIES

If at some point you have compressed your hard disk (using a product like *DoubleSpace*) it may be a good idea to reverse this. Files from the Internet are cached to your hard disk. A compressed disk will perform this task more slowly, resulting in longer on-line times and higher telephone bills.

Before doing this, however, backup all your files, and check that your hard disk will be big enough to accommodate the uncompressed files. If space is a problem consider 'zipping up' any program files you do not use that often, but do not wish to delete. Chapter 2 has details of various archiving utilities.

Configuring TCP/IP

GENERAL

Table D.1 details the data required for a typical TCP/IP configuration.

FOR WINDOWS95

Though Windows95 comes with the necessary components to connect to the Internet (TCP/IP, SLIP/PPP), it is still necessary to configure them. This section details the way I set up my connection.

Note   In this appendix commands appear in the form **Menuname I Command name**. Thus, **Settings I Control Panel** means 'click on the settings menu and then select the control panel option'.

Step 1   Check to see if dial-up networking is installed

- Click on the **My Computer** icon and see if a dial-up networking box exists. If it does, proceed to Step 2. If not, follow these instructions (you will need to have your Windows95 installation disks to hand because Windows95 will ask you to insert the disk).
- Click on **Start I Settings I Control Panel I Add/Remove Programs I Windows Setup I Communications**
- Select **Dial-up Networking** and click on **OK.** The appropriate files will be copied from the Windows95 CD-ROM or floppy disks.

Table D.1 Typical TCP/IP settings

Requirement	Example	Purpose
Your IP address	158.152.60.10	Identifies who you are
Your host name	rkiley	This combination is the text
Domain name suffix	demon.co.uk	equivalent of the IP address
Provider's name server	158.152.1.65	Converts names into numeric IP addresses
Provider's default gateway	158.152.1.65	A gateway connects two networks that would otherwise be incompatible (here, your computer to your provider's network)
Provider's subnet mask	255.255.255.0	This number, combined with your IP address identifies which network your computer is on
Protocol you are using.	PPP	Informs your provider which protocol you are using

Step 2   Install the Microsoft client

- Click on **Start** | **Settings** | **Control Panel** | **Network** | **Configuration** | **Add**
- **Network Component Type** | **Client** | **Add**
- **Manufacturer** | **Microsoft** | **Client for Microsoft networks** | **OK**

Step 3   Install the TCP/IP protocol

- Click on **Start** | **Settings** | **Control Panel** | **Network** | **Configuration** | **Add**
- **Network Component Type** | **Protocol** | **Add**
- **Manufacturer** | **Microsoft** | **TCP/IP**

Step 4   Install the dial-up adaptor

- Click on **Start** | **Settings** | **Control Panel** | **Network** | **Configuration** | **Add**
- **Network Component Type** | **Dial-up Adaptor** | **Add**
- **Network Adaptors** | **Microsoft** | **Dial-up Adaptor**

Step 5   Configure TCP/IP

- Click on **Start** | **Settings** | **Control Panel** | **Network** | **Configuration** | **TCP/IP** | **Properties**
- In **IP Address Tab**, complete your IP address and subnet mask, as supplied by *your* Internet provider (Fig. D.1).

- On the **Gateway Tab** type in the Gateway address, as supplied by *your* Internet Provider.
- On the **Bindings Tab** ensure that the **Client for Microsoft Networks** is checked.
- On the **DNS Configuration Tab** complete the **Host name**, **Domain name**, **DNS Search Server**, and **Domain suffix** as appropriate to you (Fig. D.2).

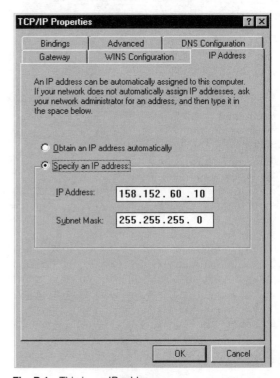

Fig. D.1   This is my IP address

- Restart *Windows95*. This will allow all these changes to take effect.

Step 6 Create a dial-up facility to call your Internet provider

- Double-click on **Dial-up Networking** icon
- Click on the **Make New Connection**, and work through the 'New Connection Wizard' (that is, supply a name for this file – I called mine 'Internet' – and the telephone number of your Internet provider).
- Click on the new **Dial-up** icon, then select **File | Properties**
- In **Server Type** check that **PPP** is selected (if you plan to use SLIP you will have to install this), and that the allowed protocol is **TCP/IP**

Step 7 Dial your provider

- Double-click your new **Dial-up** icon.
- Enter your **User name** and **Password** in the appropriate boxes, and press **Connect** (Fig. D.3).
- Your modem will dial the number, and the settings you have defined will log you on to the Internet. When connected, you will see a 'connected' screen similar to that shown in Figure D.4.
- Fire-up your Web browser, mail client etc.

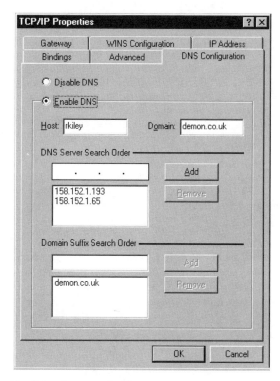

Fig. D.2 This is my DNS configuration

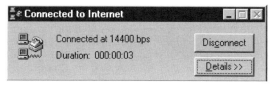

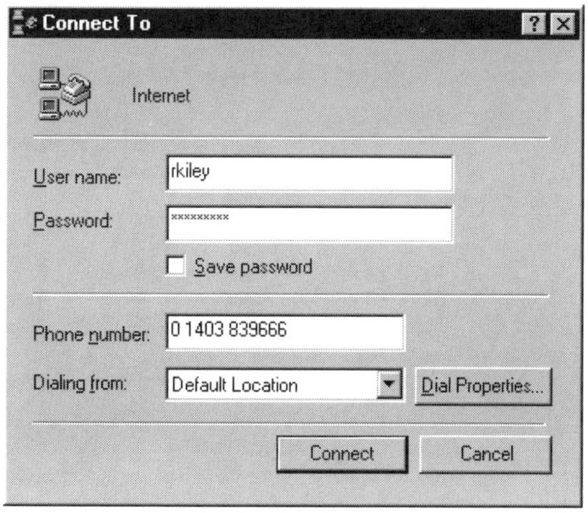

Fig. D.4 Connection acknowledgement

Fig. D.3 Connecting to the Internet

Glossary

AT command language Language used by Hayes modems and equivalents. For example, to reset your modem you can type ATZ <return>. For a complete set of commands see the documentation that came with your modem. As a rule of thumb most modems are supplied as 'Internet ready'.

BioMOO A virtual meeting place for biologists (*see also* MOOs).

bookmark Bookmarks are a way of recording the location of a particular Internet site. When you wish to revisit a book-marked site, you can do so without having to remember the specific URL.

bmp Bit mapped. A format for digitally storing an image. Alternative formats include gif and jpg.

bps Bits per second. A full page of text (in English) is approximately 16 000 bits. Thus a modem which can transmit data at 14 400 bps can send/receive the equivalent of just under one page of text per second (*see also* kbps, Mbps Gbps).

bulletin board system A computerised system that allows subscribers to post messages and exchange files.

cache A reserved space on a computer for storing items that are frequently requested. *Netscape*, for example, caches pages from the World Wide Web to the hard disk. Thus, when you want to go back to a previously accessed page, *Netscape* can retrieve it from the hard disk rather than from the original server.

client A computer program that requests the service of another computer, known as a server. Clients run on the local machine, processing and displaying information received from the server. For example, a World Wide Web browser is a client. For it to be able to do anything – such as display a page – it calls on the services of a Web server.

client software *See* client.

clock speed This refers to the speed at which the microprocessor – the 'chip' – in a computer can process information. Clock speed is measured in megahertz; the higher the number, the faster the computer can process data. An advertisement for a 'Pentium 75' means that the computer has a Pentium 'chip' with a clock speed of 75 megahertz. A 'Pentium 133' computer is, therefore, faster (and more expensive).

CU-SeeMe An Internet video conferencing facility created by Cornell University.

CU-SeeMe reflector If you wish to broadcast a conference using *CU-SeeMe* software, you must route it through a CU-SeeMe reflector. Anyone who then wants to watch the broadcast can point their *CU-SeeMe* software at the reflector. If you are using *CU-SeeMe* on a one-to-one basis you do not route this through a reflector.

data compression To speed up data transfer, most modems employ data compression facilities. The most popular of these are MNP5 and V42 bis. A modem equipped with V42 bis can multiply throughput by a factor of four. Thus, in ideal conditions a 14 400 bps modem can receive data at speeds of 57 600 bps.

dial-up A dial-up connection uses phone lines to connect one computer to another via a modem. This is the only practical way a 'home user' can connect to the Internet.

dialogue box Microsoft Windows applications use dialogue boxes as a way of communicating with you. Sometimes they may prompt you for information ('enter your search terms and press OK') and at other times they provide you with information.

DIP switches A set of switches that allows you to configure how your modem is set

when it is first switched on (*see also* AT command language).

discussion lists Subject-specific discussion groups that are participated in and distributed by e-mail. Sometimes referred to as mailing lists.

domain name The unique address of a computer on the Internet. It comprises 'sub domains' that are used to group computers together. Thus all computers with **.uk** in their domain name are located in the UK. Those which are part of the academic community are identified by the name **.ac.uk** whilst those computers located in commercial sites are assigned the name **.co.uk** (*see also* IP address).

e-mail A medium for transferring information from one location to another. This can be in the form of a text or binary file.

e-mail address An e-mail address is made up of several parts. Thus the address **abc@myplace.demon.co.uk** consists of:

user name:	**abc**
host sub-domain:	**myplace**
host name	**demon**
type of organisation	**co**
country	**uk**

e-mail signature Text that is automatically appended to every e-mail you send. Typically, this consists of your name and contact address. Good netiquette dictates that this should never be more than 3 lines long, and that pictures drawn from text characters should be avoided.

Embase A pharmacological and biomedical database consisting of more than 6 million documents. The database focuses on the pharmacological effects of drugs and chemicals.

encoded When you attach a binary file (for example, a word-processed document) to an e-mail message it is necessary to 'package' the attachment in a particular way so that the mail transport system can carry it. This is known as 'encoding' (*see also* MIME).

error correction A set of protocols used by modems to ensure that the data received matches that which was sent. If in any way the data is corrupted, it will be re-transmitted by the host server.

finger A computer program that displays information about a user (or users) currently logged-on to a local or remote system.

freenets An organisation that provides free Internet access to its 'members'. Typically, freenets are established in public libraries thus providing everyone with the opportunity to access the Internet.

FTP File transfer protocol. The most common method of moving files between Internet sites.

Gbps Gigabits per second (*see also* bps, kbps, Mbps).

gif Graphics interchange format. A graphics file format used on the Internet.

Gopher A hierarchical, menu-based system for exploring the Internet. Though this method of exploring has been completely superseded by the development of the World Wide Web, you will still encounter Gopher-based resources on your trawls of the Internet. All resources stored on Gopher servers can be accessed through a Web browser.

hard handshaking A term used to describe how modems regulate the flow of data between computers and modems to ensure data is not lost. For example, if data is transmitted more quickly than the computer can receive it, the handshaking process will send a message to the transmitter to wait. When the computer has processed that data and is ready for more, another message is sent requesting the transmission to recommence.

helper applications Helper applications extend *Netscape*'s abilities. For example, on its own *Netscape* cannot display video clips. If however, you have a client that can play video's, you can configure *Netscape* to launch this 'helper application' whenever a video appears on a Web page.

home page A starting point for Internet exploration.

host computer A host computer is one that

provides interactive services – such as Telnet and FTP – to users on the Internet.

HTML A coding language used to create hypertext documents for use on the World Wide Web. For example, to indicate that a piece of text should be displayed in bold, the text is prefixed with the code <B> and suffixed </b>. For help on authoring your own HTML pages, see the collection of resources at:

http://www.yahoo.com/Computer_ and_Internet/Internet/ World_Wide_Web/Authoring

HTTP Hypertext transfer protocol. The protocol for moving hypertext files across the Internet. Requires an HTTP client at one end, and an HTTP server at the other.

hypertext A facility that allows related documents to be linked together. Selecting a hypertext link automatically displays the related document. Thus files held on different computers (in different parts of the world) can be linked together, providing a seamless integrated information resource.

Internet provider A company or organisation that provides its clients with access to the Internet. For a fee, commercial providers allow individuals to connect their personal computers to those of the Internet provider; the provider's computers are permanently connected to the Internet.

IP address Every computer on the Internet has an IP address, known colloquially as the 'dotted quad'. An example of an IP address is 158.152.1.65. Domain names are the plain language equivalents (*see also* domain name).

ISDN terminal adaptor A device used to transmit data over a digital network in exactly the same way a modem is used to transmit data over an analogue network.

Java applet A computer program that can be included on an HTML page. When you use a Java-compatible Web browser to view a page that contains a Java applet, the applet's code is transferred to your system and executed by your browser. The Java programming language was developed by Sun Microsystems Inc. *Netscape* version 2.0 is a Java-compatible browser.

JANET Joint Academic Network. The network that links all UK higher educational establishments.

JPEG Joint photographics expert group. A file format for images. JPEG files tend to be smaller than their gif equivalents.

jpg *See* JPEG.

kbps kilobits per second (*see also* bps, Mbps, Gbps).

LINX The London Internet Exchange. A facility for existing Internet service providers to allow them to interconnect easily within the UK, and hence improve connectivity and service for their customers. Its main purpose is to avoid traffic solely between UK Internet users having to go outside the UK.

mailing lists *See* discussion groups.

MB Megabyte(s). 8 bits = 1 byte; 1 million bytes = 1 MB.

Mbps Megabits per second (*see also* bps, kbps, Gbps).

MEDLINE Incorporating the printed *Index Medicus, International Nursing Index* and the *Index to Dental Literature*, MEDLINE is the largest biomedical bibliographic database. Dating back to 1966, MEDLINE has over 7 million citations drawn from around 3600 journals.

MeSH Medical Subject Headings. The thesaurus devised by the National Library of Medicine, and used to index all articles in the MEDLINE database.

mirror To meet the demand placed on some FTP and Web sites, mirror sites were devised. As the name implies, these sites contain an exact replica of the original site. The *Netscape* FTP site is mirrored to numerous locations throughout the world. To speed up data transfer 'local' mirror sites should always be used. All things being equal, users in the UK will find that it is quicker to FTP *Netscape* from the mirror site at Imperial College, than from the main site in the US.

MIME Multi-purpose Internet mail extension. A standard for attaching non-text files (such as word-processed documents, spreadsheets etc.) to e-mail messages. An e-mail client that can send and receive attached files is said to be 'MIME compliant'.

modem Modulator demodulator. A piece of hardware that allows computers to communicate with each other through the telephone network.

MOOs Multi-user domain, object orientated. The accepted definition of a MOO is that 'it is an Internet-accessible, text-mediated virtual environment well suited for distance learning'. The easiest way to understand a MOO is to visualise it as a series of rooms, within which many individuals can congregate and interact. To move to another room you can type in cardinal directions or, if the MOO has a Web interface (like BioMOO), simply point and click to whichever room you wish to visit.

MPEG Moving picture expert group. A format for storing moving images (videos) (*see also Quicktime*).

netiquette The etiquette of the Internet. The key element in netiquette is remembering that real people are on the other end of a computer connection.

Netscape A World Wide Web browser developed by Netscape Communication Corporation.

newsgroups A worldwide system for the electronic exchange of news and views on a particular topic. Also referred to as Usenet News.

newsreader Software that is used to read messages sent to Internet newsgroups. A good newsreader will sort the messages by the subject line so that replies are shown next to the original message.

NNTP Network news transport protocol. The set of rules that dictates how Usenet News is propagated around the Internet.

NNTP server A computer (server) that you access to obtain Usenet News.

off-line Not connected. In terms of the Internet, this phrase is used to indicate that you are not connected, via the telephone line, to your Internet provider.

PING Packet Internet Gopher. PING is used to test or time the response of an Internet connection. PING sends a request to an Internet host and waits for a reply. When you PING an address, you get a response telling you the number of seconds it took to make the connection.

platform-dependent When you buy a piece of software – such as a word-processing package – you have to make sure that it its compatible with your operating system or 'platform', because software is platform-dependent. The operating system for IBM-compatible PCs is DOS or OS/2; software for these computers also usually specifies whether or not Windows is required. The operating system for Apple computers is the Macintosh System. In contrast, the Internet is *not* platform dependent. Any computer that has a copy of TCP/IP can connect to the Internet.

plug and play A term used by both hardware and software developers to describe their products. In essence it means that the product does not require any special configuring before it can be used. Open the box, plug it in, and use it. Plug and play software will typically come with an installation program that will prompt you for any necessary information.

PoP Point of presence. Most Internet providers create local points of presence to enable users to access the Internet through a local telephone number.

POP3 Post Office protocol, version 3. A set of rules designed to allow single users to read mail from a server. When e-mail is sent to you, it is stored on the server until accessed by you (*see also* SMTP).

points of presence *See* PoP.

PPP Point to point protocol. A protocol that allows dial-up users to connect to the Internet and use TCP/IP compliant clients. The alternative to PPP is SLIP.

processor size The microprocessor (or chip) is the main factor that determines how fast a computer can process data. A 386 chip is faster than a 286 but slower than a 486.

proxy server Rather than go directly to the server that hosts the data you require, you can instruct your Web browser to visit a 'proxy' server first. If the data you require is held on the proxy, it will be delivered to your desktop more quickly than from the original host. If the data is not present on the proxy, then the Web browser will automatically request the data from the host server. If your Internet provider supports 'proxy servers', I would recommend configuring your Web browser to access them (Appendix B).

public reflector *See* CU-SeeMe reflectors.

query box An on-screen form through which you can input queries. Internet search engines have query boxes where you can enter the subject for which you are searching.

Quicktime A format for storing moving images (videos) developed by Apple (*see also* MPEG).

RAM Random access memory. An allocation of space where the computer *temporarily* places software applications and the operating system for high-speed access. The more you have, the faster your computer will work. Four MB of RAM is the minimum required for Windows 3.1, whilst 8 MB of RAM is recommended for Windows95.

relevance feedback The process of using a document, retrieved from an initial search, to further refine your search. That is, once a relevant document has been found, you instruct the server to find 'more of the same'.

robots Computer programs that scour the Internet looking for new resources to index, and checking that previously identified sites are still available. Retrieved data is added to an Internet database. These databases can be interrogated using a search engine.

search engines A computer program that will undertake a search of an Internet database based on the information you have supplied.

server A computer that provides a service to client software running on other computers.

shielded modem cable The cable that connects the modem to the computer should be encased in a braid or aluminium foil. This ensures that electrical frequencies from other appliances do not interfere with the data transmission process.

SLIP Serial line Internet protocol. A protocol for using a telephone line (a serial line) and a modem to connect a computer to the Internet (*see also* PPP, TCP/IP).

SMTP Simple mail transfer protocol. A protocol used to transfer e-mail between computers.

sound card A piece of hardware in the computer that allows the user to hear computerised audio clips via external speakers.

subject catalogues An Internet subject catalogue indexes the resources of the Internet into broad subject areas, in the fashion of a library.

SuperJANET The high-speed optical computer network developed for the academic community in the UK.

T1 line A very fast data line. Capable of transmitting/receiving 1 544 000 bits per second. In pages of A4 text, this is equivalent to just under 100 pages per second.

TCP/IP Transmission control protocol/Internet protocol. Protocols that provide the basic transport mechanism for sending and receiving data on the Internet. Without TCP/IP you *cannot* connect to the Internet.

telemedicine The use of electronic means to deliver health care to persons at some distance from the provider.

Telnet An Internet service that allows your computer to directly connect, and interact with a remote computer.

uniform resource locator A way of specifying the Internet access method and location for any file or document held on the Internet.

Locators consist of three parts. Thus the URL **http://www.who.ch/wer/werindex.html** means:

http:// access method – in this case, the hypertext transport protocol
www.who.ch/ the address of server
wer/werindex.html the directory path and file name (i.e. where the file is on the server).

URL *See* uniform resource locator.

Usenet News *See* newsgroups.

UNIX An operating system designed specifically to let many people access the same computer simultaneously.

virtual reality A computer-generated simulation of a real environment. Thus, in a virtual reality environment the computer can generate visual, auditory or other sensual inputs whilst the user can interact and directly manipulate objects within this virtual world.

virus A computer virus is a computer program that has a malicious intent and that can infect other computer programs by modifying them in such a way as to include a copy of itself. The term is used loosely to cover any sort of program that tries to hide its malicious function and tries to spread onto as many computers as possible.

waiting for host to respond A message displayed by *Netscape Navigator*. It means that the Internet server you are trying to contact is not responding. As a rule of thumb, if you do not get a response within a minute, it is best to sever the connection and try again another time.

World Wide Web A global system that links information on the Internet through hypertext links embedded in documents. World Wide Web documents can contain graphics, moving images and sound.

World Wide Web browser Client software that can display any file that has been created using the hypertext markup language (HTML).

Index